An Unmitigated Disaster

An Unmitigated Disaster

America's Response to COVID-19

Robert O. Schneider

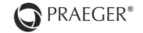 PRAEGER®

An Imprint of ABC-CLIO, LLC

Santa Barbara, California • Denver, Colorado

Library of Congress Cataloging-in-Publication Data

Names: Schneider, Robert O., author.
Title: An unmitigated disaster : America's response to COVID-19 / Robert O. Schneider.
Description: Santa Barbara, California : Praeger, [2022] | Includes bibliographical references and index.
Identifiers: LCCN 2021023960 (print) | LCCN 2021023961 (ebook) | ISBN 9781440878930 (hardcover) | ISBN 9781440878947 (ebook)
Subjects: LCSH: COVID-19 (Disease)—Political aspects—United States. | COVID-19 (Disease)—Social aspects—United States.
Classification: LCC RA644.C67 S36 2022 (print) | LCC RA644.C67 (ebook) | DDC 362.1962/414—dc23
LC record available at https://lccn.loc.gov/2021023960
LC ebook record available at https://lccn.loc.gov/2021023961

ISBN: 978-1-4408-7893-0 (print)
     978-1-4408-7894-7 (ebook)

26 25 24 23 22   1 2 3 4 5

This book is also available as an eBook.

Praeger
An Imprint of ABC-CLIO, LLC

ABC-CLIO, LLC
147 Castilian Drive
Santa Barbara, California 93117
www.abc-clio.com

This book is printed on acid-free paper ∞

Manufactured in the United States of America

Contents

Prologue

Dr. George Diaz, an infectious diseases physician in Seattle, received a phone call from the Centers for Disease Control and Prevention (CDC) on the afternoon of January 20, 2020. The CDC informed him that it had just recorded a positive test for a new strain of coronavirus in a thirty-five-year-old man who had recently returned to Washington State from Wuhan, China. The CDC also informed Dr. Diaz that it wanted to bring the patient to his hospital for treatment.

Dr. Diaz was in all probability not surprised with this news. He knew about the new coronavirus that had emerged in China and begun to circle the globe. He had to know this new virus would soon make its way to the United States. In fact, just two weeks previously, he and his hospital (Providence Regional Medical Center Everett, just outside of Seattle) had staged a tabletop drill that ran through the steps to be taken in caring for a patient with this new coronavirus. One would thus be correct in suspecting that the news just received from the CDC was not at all unexpected by Dr. Diaz or the hospital.[1]

Upon arrival at Providence Regional, the patient would be kept in an isolation room, with only the nursing staff allowed to enter. Dr. Diaz communicated with his new patient through an intercom. On his fifth day in the hospital, the patient developed pneumonia. This was a serious development. Early indications from China suggested that an alarming and disproportionate number of patients infected with the new virus who developed pneumonia were dying. Dr. Diaz was aware of a new but untried antiviral medication, remdesivir, that he thought might be applicable to this new coronavirus. Having no other proven treatment options for the new virus, he proceeded to infuse the patient with the antiviral. Within the next twenty-four hours, the patient started to feel better. As he continued to improve, the patient was soon allowed to go home under supervision. He would, in time, recover fully.

The first confirmed case of COVID-19 in the United States had been successfully treated. It was a genuine triumph of medical science. Dr. Diaz and the hospital staff had dealt with a terrifying new disease. They had responded admirably with discipline, logic, and imagination. And most importantly of all, they had achieved the best of all possible outcomes. All had gone very well indeed for patient one in the United States. Tragically, the same could not be said for every American patient who would be stricken with this new virus that swept the globe in 2020.[2]

The numbers tell the story. Between January 20, 2020, and January 29, 2021, the United States experienced 25.98 million cases of COVID-19 and recorded 433,340 deaths. Many more deaths would come in the months ahead. The year 2020 revealed to Americans—the thoughtful ones at least—some very disturbing things about their nation and themselves. Few likely understood what the first reports of a new coronavirus in China, first reported on New Year's Eve, would mean to them in the months to come. Even if they had suspected that a global pandemic was about to become a reality, few would have suspected the dramatic and tragic impact it would have on their lives and the lives of their loved ones. But the experts knew, and, theoretically, our national leaders should have known. Indeed, what was about to happen, a major public health emergency of historic proportions, was not something unexpected. It was something for which the United States had been preparing for quite some time. The previous fifteen years had seen significant effort dedicated to improving the nation's ability to respond to the threat of a global pandemic.

Nothing kills as many people in so short a time as a global pandemic. History has confirmed this time and time again. The case for pandemic preparedness is, for those who understand the nature of the threat and the inevitability of the next pandemic, a compelling one. The first line of defense against any deadly disease outbreak is to spend the resources and the time necessary to reinforce our capabilities, such as disease surveillance, diagnostic laboratories, infection control, and vaccine development. These sorts of things are more effective at containing a virus—and cost less—than waiting for an outbreak to occur and only then trying to contain it.

Yet, the United States had really not invested nearly enough in pandemic preparedness. For that matter, the global community had not invested nearly enough in pandemic preparedness. It seems that it is always easier to find money to respond to a crisis than it is to prepare for one. Be that as it may and given that more should have been done to prepare, it would not be accurate to suggest that the United States was totally unprepared for what 2020 would bring.

Since 2005 and the rapidly growing concerns about the potential for a major global pandemic, one along the lines of the 1918 Spanish flu pandemic, U.S. infectious disease experts and national leaders had engaged in major planning efforts to improve the capacity of the United States to anticipate and respond to a major pandemic crisis. Under the presidential administrations of George W. Bush and Barack Obama, one a Republican and one a Democrat, respectively, significant progress had been made in advancing the nation's preparedness. A national plan was developed, and a national response strategy was evolving. Despite the progress that had been made, there was still room for much needed improvement in the planning and for more significant funding of public health initiatives. There was understandable concern expressed by many experts that the United States, despite its significant ongoing efforts, was not nearly as well prepared for a major public health disaster as it should be. That was a concern also shared by this author in his previous work on the study of pandemic preparedness.[3,4] It is this concern that led to the writing of this book.

The pages to follow chronicle the path of the COVID-19 pandemic from January 2020 to January 2021. The narrative that unfolds will follow the month-by-month and week-by-week experience of the United States and the American people as they lived (and in too many instances died) during the unfolding of a public health crisis that as the year progressed became a truly unmitigated disaster. The first chapters set the stage for this narrative. The nature of the new virus and its emergence as a pandemic of historic proportions will be explained. An assessment of American efforts to enhance its preparedness for pandemic threats will be provided to give some context for evaluating the American 2020 response to COVID-19. The cultural and political contexts that would influence the American response, and not for the better, will be discussed as well. The details of the American response during 2020 will be shown to have constituted the story of a great failure, perhaps the greatest and most deadly failure in the nation's history.

The failure of the U.S. response to COVID-19 in 2020 was an all-too-human failure. The United States may not have had the perfect plan or the best preparation for what ultimately came to its shores with the new and deadly virus, but it did have the knowledge, resources, and capacity to do a much better job in responding to what came its way. The story of both how and why this knowledge, these resources, and this capacity were not intelligently employed in a national strategy to contain the spread of the virus and to save lives is the tale of a monumental and historic failure that should not be forgotten or forgiven. The combination of factors that contributed to the American failure to contain the spread of the virus and that allowed the pandemic to rage out of control through all of 2020 need to be understood. They need to be understood by those who lived through that dreadful year and by the generations to come. There will be other pandemics, public health disasters, and global crises in the years to come. There must never be another failure to respond like the one Americans both endured and participated in during the year 2020.

To be fair, nearly every country struggled to contain the spread of COVID-19, and they all made mistakes along the way. But one country, the United States, stood alone as the only affluent nation to have suffered severe and sustained outbreaks for the entire year in 2020. Two general factors, one cultural and the other political, account for America's great failure. On the cultural side, the United States has a tradition of prioritizing individualism over government policy action and guidance. This tradition is one of the primary reasons the United States suffers from an unequal health care system that has long produced worse medical outcomes (e.g., higher infant mortality and diabetes rates and lower life expectancy) than most other wealthy countries. In other words, Americans do not work well together. They have a deep distrust toward government and a go-it-alone mentality that eschews social cooperation.

National skepticism about government and collective action was bound to make an efficient national response to a public health crisis difficult. This difficulty was magnified by the political variables at play in the United States in 2020. These political variables contributed most to the "big fail" of 2020. In no other high-income country, and in only a few countries period, had political leaders departed from expert scientific advice as frequently and significantly as did American leaders. In no other high-income country was there such a total absence of a coordinated national response as was the case in the United States. In no other high-income country did the pandemic become quite as intensely and irrationally debated as a partisan political issue as it did in the United States.

The leaders of most countries sought to unite their citizens and prepare them to withstand the pandemic assault. This included the encouraging of collective sacrifice through the implementation of social distancing and hygiene protocols, closures, lockdowns, quarantines, and other public health measures as needed. U.S. leaders, especially the president, were reluctant to be proactive in implementing such protocols. Indeed, they seemed to politicize the pandemic rather that respond to it. This meant that instead of pulling together, Americans would find themselves drifting further apart. An already divided nation slipped into a deeper polarization at a time when unity was essential. As a result of stunningly poor (inept, actually) national leadership, the U.S. response to the pandemic was lethargic and inconsistent. In addition to its failure to follow the basic precepts of the pandemic planning that had taken place over the previous two decades, the national leadership seemed at times all too willing to dismiss the nation's best minds in science and medicine. At times, they actually worked to undermine or muzzle experts' advice. To see how all of this could have happened, and to fully comprehend its impact, is essential to even begin to understand the depth and tragedy of America's big fail in 2020. Once that is understood, those who are responsible for the big fail must be held accountable in the pages of history.

This book is but a first draft, a real-time assessment and reaction to the events of a historic year. The years to come will provide greater depth and more detail as the number of studies and publications multiply. But Americans must immediately begin to take stock. They cannot return to normal (or more likely a "new normal") without doing so. In living through what was arguably the most tumultuous year in memory, Americans must not forget the ground they have traveled over. They must not neglect to gather up the experiences of this year and apply the lessons learned.

The pages that follow will demonstrate that the United States squandered opportunity after opportunity to control the spread of the coronavirus. Despite its considerable advantages, immense resources, biomedical might, and scientific expertise, the United States floundered for a full year. The pandemic was an unmitigated disaster. The nation failed on many levels. In one year, over 430,000 died and over 25 million became sick. The breadth and magnitude of America's errors in 2020 may be difficult to fathom for many, but a virus humbled and humiliated the world's most powerful nation. It did not have to happen, and it must never happen again. This book is intended to begin gathering up the experiences and applying the lessons of 2020. It is a task that will take generations to complete, but it must begin here and now.

CHAPTER ONE

COVID-19 Makes "It" Real

We are facing a human crisis unlike any we have experienced.
—Amina J. Mohammed, UN deputy-secretary general

After all it really is all of humanity that is under threat during a pandemic.
—Margaret Chan, former director-general of the World Health
Organization

Introduction

The first recorded case appeared on November 17, 2019. This was in the Hubei Province of China. While not recognized at that time, it was the beginning of a global crisis. Eight more cases appeared in early December, with researchers pointing to an unknown virus. It would soon be identified as a new coronavirus strain that had not been previously found in humans. Symptoms included respiratory distress, fever, and cough, and in severe cases, this would lead to pneumonia and death. Like SARS, it was thought to be spread through droplets from sneezes or coughs. The new virus appeared to be very easily transmissible from human to human.

Soon, in early January 2020, the news had begun to spread that the Chinese government had locked down the city of Wuhan, where the first cases were observed, and allowed no one to enter or leave. As the world was just beginning to learn of the new coronavirus strain, ophthalmologist Dr. Li Wenliang defied Chinese government orders and released dire warnings about the new virus as he sought to provide safety information to other doctors who were treating patients with the new disease. China informed the World Health Organization (WHO) about the novel disease, but it also arrested and charged Dr. Li with a crime. Li himself would die from the new coronavirus infection just over a month after he had begun treating patients.

It was inevitable that the new virus would spread beyond Chinese borders. By mid-March, it had already spread globally to more than 163 countries. On February 11, the new virus was officially christened COVID-19. On March 11, 2020, the WHO announced that COVID-19 was officially a global pandemic. It had barreled through countries around the globe in just three months and had already infected over 118,000 people. And it was very clear that the spread was not anywhere near finished. It was expected to get much worse in a very short time. As of March 12, 2020, the United States had already seen 1,323 confirmed cases of COVID-19 and 38 deaths. New estimates were projecting that if aggressive efforts to mitigate were not undertaken, millions of Americans could eventually be infected with COVID-19. In just the next seven weeks, the number of cases in the United States would explode. By May 1, the number of U.S. cases exceeded 1 million (one-third of all cases in the world at that date), and the U.S. death toll exceeded 60,000. This was just the beginning. These numbers would continue to grow.

By April 21, 2020, the U.S. Centers for Disease Control and Prevention (CDC) reported that the United States had already seen an alarming spike in coronavirus infections and deaths. It was also made very clear by the CDC that the numbers would continue to grow. Even in the early weeks of the crisis, there was a growing public concern that the United States was lacking a coordinated national response to the COVID-19 pandemic. Several of the states implemented vigorous response efforts. At the same time, the federal government was perceived by many to be disorganized and inefficient in responding to the growing crisis. While the rest of the world seemed to be acting with greater urgency, the United States appeared to be stuck in neutral.

It is this perception that makes it critical to analyze and evaluate the federal response. There is historical and scientific context for doing so and political context that needs to be understood and analyzed as well. From the very beginning of the coronavirus pandemic, it was very clear that the United States would be challenged to once again do what it had done quite admirably and successfully in responding to global or national crises throughout its history. But for the first time in its history perhaps, it seemed not unreasonable to a growing number of informed observers to wonder whether the United States might fail to rise to the challenge.

In fairness, one must begin by accepting the fact that a pandemic cannot be stopped dead in its tracks. Even a perfect and coordinated national response could not have kept the virus from coming to the United States, and its impact would have challenged us beyond our capacity to prevent every tragic outcome. But it was increasingly suspected that what many soon saw as the federal government's bungling and inept decision-making over the first ten weeks of the crisis had turned a large-scale public health emergency into an unprecedented health, economic, and security disaster. But the bungling may not have been entirely the product of ineptitude. It may have also been the product of design. This is to say that conscious decisions made by governmental decision makers, beginning with the president of the United States, were not made without access to the necessary expert information and security intelligence required to make the best informed and optimal decisions for responding to the pandemic. Rather, a series of conscious decisions were made to ignore this information in the pursuit of other objectives. In other words, if the United States was ill prepared for or slow to respond to the crisis, it was because its leaders, inept though they might have been, consciously chose to be ill prepared or slow to respond. It was not because the United States lacked the knowledge, the ability, or the tools to be prepared and respond more effectively.

The primary purpose of this book is to evaluate the response of the United States to the COVID-19 pandemic. Of particular interest is the quality of pandemic planning and preparedness; the quality and effectiveness of national, state, and local response efforts; and the performance of national leaders during a public health crisis of historic proportions. To begin to assess whether the United States was well prepared or ill prepared, efficient or slow to respond, or organized or disorganized requires some work to understand the scientific, historic, and political contexts that provide the necessary background and perspective. That background and perspective will be an ongoing and important component in all that is to follow.

Not since 1918 and the Spanish flu had the world experienced a major pandemic as serious as COVID-19. As one might imagine, over the past one hundred years, much progress had been made in both the United States and globally in our preparations for and our responses to major public health crises. How well that progress informed and guided our response to the COVID-19 pandemic is not an insignificant question to be raised. In fact, it may be one of the most important questions to ask and answer when all is said and done. But before that question may be answered and any assessment of the American response effort may begin, it will be necessary to know what it is we needed to respond to and how it came to confront us in the first place. These questions of the "what" and the "how" will be the focus for the rest of this chapter. Knowing what "it" is that we had to deal with during this pandemic is the first step toward the evaluation of our response.

What Is COVID-19?

COVID-19 is a coronavirus. Coronaviruses make up a large family of viruses that can infect birds and mammals, including humans. Coronaviruses are common in different animals, but it is rare that an animal coronavirus can infect humans. Those that have infected humans are of several different kinds. Some coronaviruses infecting humans cause colds or other mild respiratory (nose, throat, lung) illnesses. These are things most people have experienced. In recent years, some coronaviruses have caused more serious diseases, including severe acute respiratory syndrome (SARS) and Middle East respiratory syndrome (MERS).[1] The name *coronavirus* refers to its appearance under the microscope. Coronaviruses look like they are covered with pointed structures that surround them like a corona, or crown.

COVID-19 was a new strain of the coronavirus not previously found in humans. Where did it come from? As already noted, the first cases were uncovered in China. As of this writing, researchers and health officials are still tracing the exact cause of this new coronavirus. An early hypothesis thought it may be linked to a seafood market in Wuhan, China. Some people who visited the market developed viral pneumonia caused by the new coronavirus. Investigations were ongoing, and would be for some time, as to how this new virus originated and spread.[2] But a picture was beginning to emerge.

The origin story of coronavirus focused on the Huanan Seafood Market in Wuhan. The first media reports noted that someone became infected with the new virus from an animal. Scientists reportedly said the virus came from bats. They noted that it was probably first passed through an intermediary animal before moving to humans. This had happened with other coronaviruses. The coronavirus that produced the 2002 SARS outbreak is an example. In that case, the virus had moved from bats to catlike civets before infecting humans.[3] While the origins of COVID-19 may not be definitively agreed upon at the time of this writing, it must be noted that most viruses that infect humans do come through animals.

One can never predict exactly which viruses will infect humans and become easily transmissible from human to human, but new virus strains that make this leap are typically the cause of major epidemics or pandemics. The highly predictable process works something like this: It starts with the migration of agriculture and urban environments into remote areas. This increases the likelihood that a new virus strain will come into contact with humans. Thanks to the increased densification of both the animal and human populations, these pathogens can spread in a localized community. If it becomes easily transmissible from human to human and is a particularly severe (perhaps deadly) virus, it may easily become the cause of greater problems. Given the frequency and the ease of modern travel, it may circulate the globe in a matter of days and fuel the beginning of a global pandemic.[4,5]

Regardless of how exactly COVID-19 was spread to humans, we know for certain that it is easily transmissible from human to human. How was it transmitted? Researchers were quickly able to tell us that the new coronavirus was spread through droplets released into the air when an infected person coughed or sneezed. The droplets generally did not travel more than a few feet, and they fell to the ground (or onto surfaces) in a few seconds. This is why social and physical distancing was proven to be effective in preventing the spread. The incubation period for COVID-19 was shown to be fourteen days. This means that symptoms could show up in people up to fourteen days after initial exposure to the virus. Given the ease of transmission, the two-week incubation period, and the fact that asymptomatic persons may carry and transmit the virus, containing its spread is difficult. Only aggressive social distancing measures can help slow the spread of a virus like COVID-19. All coronaviruses can be transmitted between humans through respiratory droplets that infected people expel when they breathe, cough, or sneeze. A typical surgical mask or other face covering cannot block out all the viral particles contained in these droplets, but using masks would soon prove to be effective in significantly reducing the spread of the virus. There were other simple measures—such as washing your hands; disinfecting frequently touched surfaces and objects; and avoiding touching your face, eyes, and mouth— that were also recommended by public health experts to reduce the risk of infection.[6]

What were the symptoms of COVID-19? These would become well known to all in a very short time as the virus became a global pandemic. Symptoms included cough, fever, shortness of breath, muscle aches, sore throat, unexplained loss of taste or smell, diarrhea, and headache. In extreme cases, COVID-19 led to severe respiratory problems, kidney failure, and, in the most severe cases, death. The early breakdown of how the symptoms progress suggested that the disease ran its course in about two weeks (see box 1.1). In the most serious cases, the average time to death was 18.5 days.

BOX 1.1 COVID-19 SYMPTOMS

Most common symptoms include
    Fever or chills
    Cough
    Shortness of breath or difficulty in breathing
    Fatigue
    Muscle or body aches
    Headache
    Loss of taste or smell
    Sore throat
    Congestion or runny nose
    Nausea or vomiting
    Diarrhea
More serious cases may experience the following
    Greater difficulty breathing
    Chest pain or pressure
    Loss of speech or of movement

Source: Centers for Disease Control and Prevention, https://www.cdc.gov/coronavirus/2019-ncov/symptoms-testing/symptoms.html

How did COVID-19 kill? This was a question initially surrounded with uncertainty that would make it difficult for researchers and doctors to determine the best way to treat critically ill patients. The uncertainty had to do with the inability to determine whether death was caused by the virus itself or by a person's own immune system. Early analysis suggested that it was not only the virus that ravaged the lungs that posed the threat of death; an overactive immune response might also make people severely ill or cause death. Early studies suggested that the immune system response had played a part in the decline and death of people infected with COVID-19. This spurred a push for treatments (steroids, for example) that rein in the immune response. But, as many feared, some of these treatments that act broadly to suppress the immune system could actually hamper the body's ability to keep the viral infection in check.

That damage might be caused by both the virus and the immune system is not uncommon. Many symptoms associated with any virus are due to the protective responses of the human immune system. The runny nose one has during a cold is not a direct effect of the virus but a result of the immune system's response to the cold virus. The fever that accompanies the cold is the immune system working to increase its efficiency in fighting off the infection. It is working to make the body less hospitable to the virus. By resting when one has these symptoms, one allows the immune system to do its thing. Social withdrawal (i.e., staying home when sick) helps decrease the spread of the virus.

Of course, one may have the virus before the symptoms appear. It must be noted that people infected with viruses such as coronavirus often do not show symptoms until several days after infection. By then, collateral damage from the immune response is likely contributing to the illness. This also means one may be contagious and spreading the virus before becoming aware of the need for treatment, rest, and social disengagement. It is very hard to precisely determine how much of the illness is due to the virus itself and what or how much is attributable to the immune response. But one can say with certainty that it is almost always a combination of the two.[7]

Among the more confounding aspects of the novel coronavirus known as COVID-19 as it spread around the world was the wide range of disease severity that patients experienced. Only a minority of COVID-19 patients would require hospitalization, but the effects of the infection for these people were very dramatic and in some cases life-threatening. Among twenty-year-olds, the hospitalization rate was about 1 percent. This rate increased to 8 percent for people in their fifties and closer to almost 19 percent for people over the age of eighty. Among diagnosed cases, the death rate was initially said to be about 3.4 percent, but this soon leveled off to about 1.4 percent.[8] The risks of severe cases and death increased with age. The risk of hospitalization was much greater for those over the age of fifty, and there was a greater proportion of cases likely to result in death than for those under fifty. Children were found to be the least likely to die, with death rates in confirmed cases of less than 1 percent in newborns to nine-year-olds. That rose to 4.28 percent in people seventy and older and to 7.8 percent for people eighty years and above.

Who was at the highest risk for severe illness? According to the CDC, those with the highest risk were sixty-five years and older. Especially at risk were senior citizens living in nursing homes or long-term facilities. People of all ages with underlying medical conditions were also at high risk. This included people with chronic lung disease or moderate to severe asthma, people with serious heart conditions, and people who were immunocompromised. Also included in the high-risk category were people with severe obesity, diabetes, chronic kidney disease, and people with liver disease.[9] Depending on where one stood on the demographic spectrum, the early assessments of risk were either alarming or somewhat reassuring. But experts were very quick to note that this disease and the global outbreak that unfolded was its own unique beast. With so much unknown, no surefire treatment, and a vaccine a good way off into the future, they all warned that the world was in uncharted territory.

COVID-19, as noted earlier, received its official name on February 11, 2020. That is when a WHO press briefing made it official. COVID-19 is an acronym. In its full form, it stands for coronavirus disease of 2019. Why was this name chosen? This was explained by the director-general of the WHO in his remarks announcing the new disease: "Under agreed guidelines between WHO, the World Organization for Animal Health and the Food and Agriculture Organization of the United Nations, we had to find a name that did not refer to a geographical location, an animal, an individual or group of people, and which is also pronounceable and related to the disease."[10] One month later, on March 11, 2020, the WHO declared COVID-19 to be a pandemic. Just what is a pandemic? Why is COVID-19 a pandemic? Knowing the answers to these questions and why they matter is something not to be taken for granted.

What Is a Pandemic?

In short, a pandemic is a global outbreak of a disease, and an epidemic refers to the sudden and rapid outbreak and spread of a disease in a localized setting or across a particular region or regions. For example, the Zika virus outbreak that began in Brazil in 2014 and made its way across the Caribbean and Latin America was an epidemic. The Ebola outbreak in West Africa in 2014–2016 was also an epidemic. The U.S. Department of Health and Human Services (HHS) considers the misuse of opioids in the United States and the number of deaths caused by this to be an epidemic. Pandemics are usually first classified as epidemics. COVID-19 began as an epidemic in China. Epidemics do not always become pandemics, but as COVID-19 made its way around the world fairly quickly, it become a pandemic. A pandemic is a novel disease that spreads around the globe, is easily transmissible because people do not have immunity to the new virus, has a high rate of infection, and may result in potentially millions of deaths.[11]

There have been pandemics in modern times that people living today may remember. Many people have lived through several. The most severe pandemic in the last one hundred years was the Spanish flu of 1918. It infected nearly one-third of the world's population and killed between 30 million and 50 million people (about a 3 percent death rate). In the United States, it infected 25 percent of the population and resulted in 675,000 deaths. The 1957–1958 Asian flu (1.1 million deaths worldwide), the 1968 Hong Kong flu (an estimated 1 million deaths worldwide), and the H1N1 swine flu of 2009–2010 (over a billion people infected worldwide but a low mortality rate) are lesser pandemics of recent vintage.[12] The point is, pandemics are not as rare as some may think. Influenza pandemics have occurred about three times every century since 1500. Not all are of equal severity, but some have changed history (see box 1.2). Civilizations may rise, but diseases also sometimes rise to strike them down.

Given the seriousness and the stakes of pandemic scenarios, the most important thing that matters is the relationship between governments and the truth. Political leaders need to understand the truth, handle the truth, convey the truth, and promote the effectiveness of those experts who know the truth. In the midst of something as serious as a global pandemic, the

---

Box 1.2   Timeline of Pandemics Throughout History

430 BCE—Earliest recorded pandemic in history

165 CE—Antonine plague (the earliest appearance of smallpox)

250—Cyprian plague

541—Justinian plague

Eleventh century—Leprosy

1350—Black Death

1492—Columbian Exchange (i.e., arrival of the Spanish in the New World)

1665—Great Plague of London

1817—First cholera pandemic

1875—Fiji measles pandemic

1889—Russian flu

1918—Spanish flu

1957—Asian flu

1981—HIV/AIDS

2003—SARS (severe acute respiratory syndrome)

Source: History.com, "Pandemics That Changed History," https://www.history.com/topics/middle-ages/pandemics-timeline

role of politics and personality must be limited, and the steps to be taken must be based on scientifically solid evidence and well-developed plans with explicit triggers for actions taken or not taken. At least, that should be the goal.

The literature on pandemics tells us a great deal about their origins, our responses to them, and the psychological impacts they may have upon us.[13–15] But of equal if not greater importance is the role of leadership during a pandemic crisis. The speed and scope of the COVID-19 crisis inevitably posed extraordinary challenges. Even under the best of circumstances, leaders in our public and private institutions would have missed opportunities to act or mitigate in a timely fashion. Some of these missed opportunities are to be expected in any crisis that emerges so quickly and unexpectedly. But it would be a mistake to think that failures of leadership are something we should expect in all crisis situations.

As a general rule, crises are not totally unexpected. They may be anticipated to some extent. Most pandemics, for example, are the predictable result of those places and circumstances where humanity and nature collide. Today, the scientific foundation exists for societies and their leaders to reasonably anticipate the viral threats on the horizon that may ignite the next pandemic. It may be difficult to impossible to identify the exact virus that will mutate and become the source of the next pandemic, but there has been enough expert analysis to conclusively warn us that the next pandemic is coming. It is never a question of if that will happen; it is always a question of when.

It can be said with certainty that the world had been preparing for the next pandemic for some time. It can also be said that as COVID-19 emerged, the world should have known exactly what to expect. As will be documented in chapter 2, there should have been no surprises in how things unfolded as the virus circled the globe. Despite the advances of modern medicine, the absence of a vaccine and the shortages of antivirals; the shortages of personal protective equipment (PPE) for doctors, nurses, and first responders; and the problems associated with rapidly accelerating transmission rates and hospital admissions were all things to be anticipated. A pandemic, it was said, would strike like a tsunami. It would inundate intensive care units, and doctors and nurses would begin to fall ill themselves. The caseload, the shortages of equipment, the lack of effective treatment options, and the health risks to health care providers were all expected to push the health care system to the point of collapse.

It was well known that a pandemic was something that would bring most hospitals to their knees. Hospitals, like every other American industry, have done everything imaginable to reduce their costs. This means a reduction in the number of hospital beds and virtually no excess capacity available for extraordinary circumstances considered unlikely to occur. On a per capita basis, the United States in 2020 had far fewer hospital beds than it had a few decades earlier. During an average flu season, the usage of respirators struggles to meet the demand. During a pandemic, it was reasonably feared that many people who needed a mechanical respirator may not have access to one.

It was equally well known that a pandemic would have a disastrous impact on the global economy. With illness spreading among workers, quarantine measures enforced to slow the spread of disease, and production lines shut down, just-in-time delivery systems and supply chains would collapse, and unemployment and worker absentee rates would both soar to historic levels. Working from home would become the new norm for many. Schools, day-care facilities, and small businesses would close down for weeks. With no vaccine and no effective antiviral drugs available for treatment, all of these things were seen as inevitable in any pandemic scenario. They were all to be expected when nature went to war with humanity and attacked it with a pandemic.

Despite all that was known and the serious work done by governments the world over to prepare for the inevitability of the next pandemic, it was a bit eerie to watch COVID-19 emerge and reach across the globe. Some compared its approach to that of a slow-moving hurricane. Of course, the technology exists today to pinpoint the path of a hurricane and indicate which of us is directly in harm's way. Our inability to know which of us might ultimately be infected with or targeted by a coronavirus that would soon impact the entire nation was much different from a hurricane whose path could be reasonably predicted. This no doubt broadened the level of concern many Americans began to feel as the pandemic storm approached. Whatever its potential impact and whatever we knew or did not know about pandemics, we did know that one was coming. And whatever it was, it was about to get very real.

As the virus circled the world, it was interesting to see how governments reacted. Many of those who responded most successfully were quick and efficient in their efforts to implement various mitigation strategies, including closures and social distancing. The United States had the relative advantage of having ten weeks to prepare as it observed the efforts of other nations in response to the pandemic. There was never any question that the United States would need to be prepared to implement defensive measures in a timely and coordinated response to what was coming its way.

The First Wave: The Global Time Line

The daily news reports, to be summarized here in an attempt to capture the building drama of the unfolding global crisis, would come to dominate the lives of all Americans. New Year's Eve is a time of reflection and a time of celebration. It frequently means bidding adieu to the disappointments of the old year and the anticipation of new beginnings and new hopes for the year to come. December 31, 2019, brought news that would come to dominate everything else that 2020 might bring. One may not have known it, but the daily news updates to follow would be dominated by the impact of the story reported on this New Year's Eve about the Huanan Seafood Wholesale Market, a wet market in the city of Wuhan. It was on this day that Chinese officials first notified the WHO of a mysterious new disease. This disease, identified as a new coronavirus, was thought to have spread through a large gathering of people at a live animal food market. It was extremely contagious and, in the most serious cases, resulted in a deadly pneumonia.

On New Year's Day, Chinese authorities closed the Huanan Seafood Wholesale Market. The Chinese government also banned the trade of live animals at all wet markets and announced a temporary national ban on the buying, selling, and transportation of wild animals in markets, restaurants, and online marketplaces across the country. This ban was later made permanent. On January 7, 2020, Chinese authorities identified the virus that caused the pneumonia-like illness as a new type of coronavirus. On January 11, China recorded its first death linked to the novel coronavirus, a sixty-one-year-old man who had been a frequent customer at the Huanan market.

January 13, 2020, saw the first case of coronavirus outside of China. This was in Thailand, where a sixty-one-year-old female tourist was diagnosed. She had recently spent time in Wuhan, China. In response to this report, airports in Hong Kong, Singapore, Thailand, and South Korea began to closely screen all passengers for fever. One week later, on January 20, the first U.S. case was reported in Snohomish County, Washington. This first case on American soil was a thirty-five-year-old man who had been evacuated from Wuhan, China, and landed back at the Seattle–Tacoma International Airport on January 15. Though he initially showed no symptoms, he reported to an urgent care clinic with symptoms of pneumonia on January 19. He was diagnosed with the new coronavirus a day later.

On January 23, China placed the city of Wuhan under quarantine. A few days later, all of Hubei Province was placed under quarantine. This meant the full lockdown of over sixty million people, the largest quarantine in history. On January 30, the WHO declared an international health emergency. The next day, January 31, President Donald Trump banned foreign nationals (but not returning U.S. citizens) from entering the United States if they had been in China within two weeks prior. On February 2, the first COVID-19 death outside of China was announced. This case was recorded in the Philippines.

On February 7, Li Wenliang, a Wuhan doctor and coronavirus whistleblower, died. Dr. Li's death came a little more than a month after he had sent out a warning message to other doctors. In that message, he had described his experiences working with patients exhibiting troubling pneumonia-like symptoms at the hospital where he worked. For this, Wuhan police arrested Li, and he was forced to sign a letter saying he was making false comments. By February 9, the coronavirus death toll in China had surpassed that of the 2002–2003 severe acute respiratory syndrome (SARS) epidemic, which killed about 774 people globally. The new coronavirus killed nearly three times as many people in eight weeks than SARS did in eight months. On February 11, the WHO announced that the disease caused by the new coronavirus would be called "COVID-19."

By February 12, news reports suggested that the number of China's new cases had begun to stabilize. But it was also on this day that coronavirus cases started to spike in South Korea. The Korean government believed that the spike may have ignited due to a large gathering at a church. The tightly packed services had become super-spreader events by the Korean CDC's reckoning. South Korea would proceed aggressively. It implemented widespread testing as a response measure. The country soon began conducting as many as ten thousand tests per day, and drive-through testing clinics were built where the tests could detect coronavirus cases in just ten minutes. Officials said the clinics were able to reduce testing time by a third. By April 1, South Korea had tested more than 420,000 people for the new coronavirus and confirmed nearly ten thousand cases.

Valentine's Day (February 14, 2020) brought news of Europe's first death associated with the COVID-19 outbreak. A Chinese tourist who had tested positive for the virus died in France. February would also bring news of a serious outbreak in Iran. With 18,400 confirmed coronavirus cases, Iran was the third most affected country after China and Italy. All of the country's schools and universities were closed down on February 23 along with many movie theaters and cultural centers. Neighboring countries Turkey and Pakistan also closed their borders with Iran. Twenty-three members of the Iranian Parliament had become infected with the virus, and one had died. Some reports accused the Iranian government of censoring the media and covering up the true scope of the outbreak. This, of course, is exactly what should never be done during a public health emergency.

On February 21, the number of COVID-19 cases spiked dramatically in Italy. This signaled a serious outbreak in the country. With 110,000 infected, Italy overtook China as the nation with the most coronavirus cases reported. Italy also had the world's highest death toll at more than 13,000. News reports and scenes on American television screens showed grim insights into what a pandemic might look like. February 29 brought news of the first confirmed death from COVID-19 on American soil. The first publicly confirmed U.S. death related to the coronavirus was a man in his fifties with chronic underlying health issues. He died at a hospital in King County, Washington. Between February 29 and March 19, nearly all U.S. states had declared a state of emergency. These declarations would help states activate emergency response plans and spend more money on preparedness actions. Such declarations also authorized leaders to use funds to deploy additional personnel, buy equipment, and prepare stockpiles.

On March 3, coronavirus cases spiked sharply in Spain, signifying the start of an outbreak. By March 31, Spain would have over one hundred thousand cases and nine thousand deaths, the world's second-highest death toll up to that time. On March 9, Italy placed all sixty million of its citizens on lockdown. Initially, two regions near Milan and Venice in the north became hot spots for cases; they were locked down on February 23. The country's leadership shut down schools, museums, and public venues and discouraged large gatherings. By March 9, the government had expanded the coronavirus restriction zone to encompass the entire nation. All stores closed except for grocery markets and pharmacies. The entire country was on lockdown.

On March 11, the WHO officially declared the COVID-19 global outbreak to be a pandemic. The geographic spread of the disease, the severity of the illness it caused, and its effects on society had reached the point that the reality of a global pandemic could no longer be doubted. On this same day, President Trump announced a ban on travel from twenty-six European countries. The United Kingdom and Ireland were later added. However, the ban did not stop U.S. citizens from reentering the country from Europe. On March 13, President Trump finally declared a national emergency. This declaration triggered the release of federal aid to states, municipalities, and U.S. territories. A few days later, in a leaked one hundred–page federal document reported in the *New York Times*, the nation would become aware of just how dire the situation might be. The document noted that product shortages impacting health care, emergency services, and other elements of critical infrastructure could exacerbate things considerably. It warned of expected shortages with respect to staffing, diagnostic capabilities, and medical supplies, including PPE and pharmaceuticals, until an effective vaccine was developed. As early as January, the WHO had recommended that all nations prepare for containment, active surveillance, early detection, isolation, case management, contact tracing, and prevention of the spread of the coronavirus. This report suggested that the United States may not have taken that recommendation to heart.

By March 23, New York City had become the epicenter of the coronavirus epidemic in the United States. With nearly 21,000 cases (mostly persons under the age of sixty) already confirmed, the expectation was that the city was about to experience a very severe outbreak. By March 26, the United States was the world leader in confirmed cases. On that date, it had 82,404 confirmed cases, surpassing China's 81,782 and Italy's 80,589. It was also very clear that these numbers would continue to increase. On April 2, with over a third of the global population under some form of lockdown, the world passed the 1 million mark in COVID-19 infections.

As coronavirus cases grew within the nation's borders, the federal government was incredibly slow to act. Against the advice of almost all medical experts, it was relying on travel restrictions to prevent the virus from entering the country. It neither anticipated any serious outbreaks nor provided any direction for mitigation. Alone among the nations of the world, the United States seemed to have no national strategy, and it appeared to be much slower to implement defensive measures to slow the spread of the disease.

Lacking clear guidance from the federal government, the governors of several states began to take more aggressive steps as the caseloads mounted. They took the unprecedented steps of issuing "stay-at-home" orders. This meant that residents would avoid going out into public places except for essential services, and they could go to work in the critical sectors that would remain open. California Governor Gavin Newsom issued the first statewide stay-at-home order on March 19. Other states would soon follow suit. By April 7, about 95 percent of all Americans were under some form of partial lockdown as a result of state, county, or city orders.

By April 10, the global death toll associated with COVID-19 had topped one hundred thousand. By April 15, the global number of confirmed cases had reached two million. It had increased from one million to two million in just five days. By April 11, the economic impact of the pandemic had become painfully visible as the number of Americans who had filed for unemployment had reached twenty-two million. In just four weeks, from mid-March to mid-April, coronavirus-associated layoffs had erased more than a decade of record job creation in the United States. In the midst of these rapidly alarming developments in the United States, President Trump ordered a halt on $400 million in U.S. funding for the WHO. He blamed the WHO for not sharing information in a timely fashion and suggested that this was one of the primary reasons the pandemic had spread before nations were ready to address it. Most experts wondered how ending the U.S. annual contribution to the WHO would improve anything. They also warned that this defunding by the United States might mean that the pandemic could last for many more months, even years, longer.

By April 19, the American media was flooded with stories and scenes of protesters holding anti-lockdown rallies. In state after state, protesters assembled with signs, semiautomatic weapons, and anger to express their opposition to the restrictions placed upon them by the stay-at-home orders. Reporting from multiple news outlets found links between many of these protests and President Donald Trump's reelection campaign. The president himself tweeted his support for the protests and urged his followers to "liberate" the various states where governors (primarily Democratic governors) had been too aggressive, as he perceived it. While this spectacle unfolded and was exhaustively covered, opinion surveys nevertheless showed overwhelming public support for the stay-at-home orders.

On April 21, a person in California was found to have died from COVID-19 on February 6, three weeks earlier than what authorities had previously figured was the first American pandemic death. The autopsies of three people who had died in their homes between February 6 and February 17 indicated the deceased had tested positive for coronavirus. It had been thought that the first American death from coronavirus had occurred in Washington State on February 29. These three deaths in Northern California indicated that the first American death had occurred three weeks earlier. The next day, April 22, the United States reported the highest single-day death toll, over twenty-six hundred, for any country.

On April 27, the White House rolled out its blueprint for reopening the economy. It included ramping up coronavirus testing programs. This was considered essential for a safe reopening of the economy. The networks and the print media reported that the federal government would be prepared to send enough diagnostic tests to the states to screen about 2 percent of their populations. This would amount to two hundred thousand tests per day, which was about five hundred times lower than independent analysts were calling for at the time. At this rate, it would take four years to test every American. As the month of May began, and with both case numbers and deaths still on the rise in many parts of the nation, the push to reopen the economy and to end the state shutdowns was in full swing and moving forward.

On May 20, 2020, the CDC update reported the United States had tallied 1,528,661 cases of COVID-19 and 91,938 deaths. These numbers would continue to increase, of course. American deaths would soon top 100,000. With 4 percent of the world's population, the United States had experienced almost one-third of the cases and deaths associated with the pandemic through its first wave. As of May 20, 323,300 people had died of COVID-19 worldwide. Confirmed infections stood at 4.9 million in 188 countries and territories. Nearly 1.7 million people had recovered from the disease by May 20. Looking at these numbers, or looking at a nation-by-nation breakdown of the top tallies across the globe (see table 1.1), may give rise to some interesting questions.

In addition to the largest number of cases and deaths of any nation, almost one-third of the global total up to May 20, the United States had

Table 1.1   Top 15 Nations—COVID-19 Cases and Deaths (May 20, 2020)

	Nation	Cases	Deaths
1.	United States	1,528,661	91,938
2.	Russia	299,941	2,837
3.	Brazil	271,885	17,983
4.	United Kingdom	250,138	35,422
5.	Spain	232,037	27,778
6.	Italy	226,699	32,169
7.	France	180,933	28,025
8.	Germany	177,827	8,112
9.	Turkey	151,615	4,199
10.	Iran	124,603	7,119
11.	India	106,886	3,303
12.	Peru	99,483	2,914
13.	China	84,063	4,638
14.	Canada	80,498	6,028
15.	Saudi Arabia	59,854	329

Source: Johns Hopkins University, https://coronavirus.jhu.edu/map.html (see for daily updates)

the eleventh-highest death rate out of more than 140 countries tracked by Johns Hopkins University. The United States was averaging 28.1 deaths per 100,000 people.[16] Differences in mortality rates can be accounted for by the differences in the number of people tested. With more testing, more people with milder cases are identified. This would lower the case-to-fatality ratio. Since the United States was lagging far behind in its testing capacity, the death rate may have been lower. Demographic factors were also a factor. For example, the coronavirus death rate will be higher for older people and people with preexisting conditions. It is also very important to note that characteristics of the health care system matters a great deal. For example, mortality may rise as hospitals become overwhelmed and have fewer resources. Other factors, to be discussed in subsequent chapters, may also come into play.

As the number of new coronavirus cases confirmed in the United States was beginning to show a modest decline in mid-May, optimistic reports were saying that the United States was just passing the peak of daily deaths related to the virus. This suggested we were now in a slow downward phase of daily deaths. After five months of intense worry and stay-at-home orders, and eager to reopen the economy, this was welcome news for most Americans. But it did not signify the end of worry or an end to the pandemic. Even as things began to slowly reopen, it was projected that the raw number of deaths would increase. By August 1, according to Institute for Health Metrics and Evaluation at the University of Washington, the United States would top 134,000 deaths. (It would actually be more, as the death toll had topped 150,000 by that date.) Even under the best of circumstances, one had to know that the future would be tenuous and uncertain as the nation reopened its economy. Reopening the economy too quickly could result in a massive return of infections. Expected spikes could turn into new outbreaks if states did not have in place the capability to respond to these spikes when they appeared. Also, and of great importance, the nation had to be prepared for an inevitable second wave of the pandemic in the fall or winter.

Just as the first five months of 2020 were in many respects a nightmare, there was reason to suspect that we had not yet seen the whole of it. The historic pandemic, the worst in over one hundred years, was a constant dark and foreboding cloud lurking over every moment of every day. But these five months were just a beginning, and we had to know it. Coronavirus was not about to cease to be a concern, and the road ahead was as uncertain as ever, even as hope for better days ahead seemed to be on the rise with the approach of summer. Unfortunately, this would turn out to be a false hope.

Conclusion: "It" Must be Understood

As the events of the first five months of 2020 unfolded—as a pandemic of historic proportions unraveled our daily routines and activities faster than we could ever have imagined—we could be forgiven if we might have wondered whether life as we knew it would ever be the same again. After the whirlwind of pandemic news and developments coming at us daily as the coronavirus circled the globe, we could also be forgiven if we did not exactly comprehend what was happening, why it was happening, or what to expect next. We had all heard the word *pandemic* before, but did we really know what that meant? For at least the last couple of decades, warnings of a pandemic were often ignored despite the mounting evidence that all nations needed to have some urgency about preparing for one. It was not at all unreasonable to ask ourselves, as nature was dramatically imposing new risks upon humanity, "Are we ready for this?"

Many experts, as shall be demonstrated in chapter 2, had warned that a major pandemic was an inevitability for the near future. The science was producing the evidence, and the risks were identifiable and growing. Of course, one could not predict when a specific virus would mutate, when it would become transmissible from human to human, or when it would ignite a global pandemic, but the number of risks were easily identifiable and were growing. As this evidence mounted, the nations of the world did commit to more pandemic planning and preparedness. But was it enough?

To many experts, it did not seem to be enough. The suspicion was that the arc of a future pandemic would be predictable, and not in an encouraging way. People would deny or dismiss a threat until it became impossible to ignore. Governments would not have stockpiled sufficient protective equipment and supplies to respond effectively. There would be no vaccine or antiviral medications available to respond. Governments would be slow to react and would not always follow the science. The only weapons available to confront a pandemic would be social distancing and stay-at-home orders. These drastic measures would, if implemented in a timely and effective way, be valuable weapons against a pandemic virus. They would also have some dramatic economic side effects. The public, cooperative at first, would too quickly grow weary of restrictions and precautions. This could quite possibly lead to a tragic underestimation of the deadly course that a pandemic might ultimately take. All of this was yet to play out as the year 2020 began, but everything to come should have been anticipated. It was all quite predictable, but were we really prepared?

The thought that the United States might not have been prepared for the coronavirus pandemic should not be regarded as a controversial thought. The United States has been unprepared before, and well within recent memory. The United States and its leaders were surprised and unprepared when terrorists hijacked airplanes and attacked the homeland on September 11, 2001. The financial crisis of 2008 was totally predictable but still unexpected by public- and private-sector leaders. The devastation from Hurricane Andrew in Florida in 1992 and Hurricane Katrina in New Orleans in 2005 exposed serious gaps in the government's disaster response and emergency management systems. But none of these failings were really a surprise when one examines them in detail.

Various crises have shown that the government of the United States is rarely, if ever, fully prepared. Even when it has planned for a crisis, it is difficult for government to be as flexible as it needs to be to respond as quickly and creatively as crisis conditions typically demand. Many factors contribute to what might be called the chronic weaknesses in our preparedness for disasters. Preparing for a future crisis or disaster, even when attempted in good faith and with the proper tools, always falls short of the mark. Part of the reason is that preparing for and committing significant resources to preparing for something that might happen at some imprecisely defined future time is a hard sell. The pressing needs of the moment always seem to be more important and become an excuse for not committing scarce resources and valuable time to something seen (incorrectly) as unpredictable or of low probability. Even when a crisis teaches us of the need to think differently and to prepare for the future, there is a tendency to focus on the lessons learned after the last crisis. As a result, our government tends to be reactive. It reacts to a crisis rather than preparing for one. This often ensures the failure of the response, as it allows the crisis to inundate and become catastrophic before a response can even begin.

Preparation for any crisis, including a pandemic, must mean above all else planning ahead. It means putting the organization and the structures in place that will guide decision-making as a crisis begins to unfold. But even if there is a plan in place, no one can really be as fully prepared for a crisis as they would like to be. No plan will be perfect because each crisis confronts us with unexpected twists. A good plan can minimize chaos, especially at the beginning, and ensure that government is agile enough to figure out what to do next. The U.S. government does plan. It had plans for a pandemic. But, as already noted, planning is not always a priority that is supported or done with consistency. Planning for the next crisis takes money. Political leaders are often reluctant to spend that money or, at the very least, are unwilling to spend as much of it as they should to plan for the next crisis. They have other competing priorities that they deem as more important and more immediate. Even if the money is available, it is never enough, and the political battles over determining how to spend it can defeat the purpose of spending it.

A quick scan of the time line for the first wave of the COVID-19 pandemic, as presented in this chapter, does not begin to answer many questions we may have pondered as we lived it. Were we prepared? We had at least two solid months' warning. Was this time used to our best advantage? How could it have been better used? Why, with 4 percent of the world's population, did the United States suffer a disproportionate one-third of the global cases in the early months? Why was the death toll in the United States so much greater than the rest of the world? What was the nature of our national response, and how well did it work? How well did our national, state, and local leadership function as the crisis unfolded? Did our experiences in the first wave help us to be better prepared for future waves or spikes in infections? These are the some of the questions that we need to answer before we can begin to reasonably evaluate the American response to the COVID-19 pandemic.

In the pages to follow, we begin with an examination of U.S. pandemic planning and preparedness activity over the past couple decades. From there, we proceed to an examination of the political and cultural context in which that planning occurred and which would almost certainly influence how both the U.S. government and its citizens responded to the crisis. A detailed examination of the national response to the first wave of the pandemic and an examination of how the American public responded follow. The impact of subsequent spikes in infections throughout the year is then assessed, with a particular focus on how well the lessons of the first wave were applied.

The coronavirus pandemic, like all pandemics, would be a long-term and ongoing crisis to be dealt with. Until an effective vaccine was developed, something that typically takes considerable time, and readily available to all citizens, Americans (and all of humanity) would live in a coronavirus world. We would continue to assess risks for an extended time. Can we go back to work? Can we go to a restaurant or bar? Can we go to the beach? Can children go back to school? Can we visit Grandma? A return to anything approximating normal would be a long, drawn-out matter. Even after the pandemic ends, human society will be changed in some dramatic ways, for better or worse. Its impact will never vanish completely for anyone who has lived through it. Many Americans recall 9/11 and the 2008 financial crisis as events that reshaped American society in some lasting ways. All major disasters or crises have that sort of impact. There can be no doubt that the COVID-19 pandemic will one day be recalled for its lasting impact on the reshaping of our society. But before we can begin to speculate about or assess any of that, we must understand what has happened. That understanding will be necessary to ensure that the long-term societal changes to come are for better and not for worse.

The first question to be answered is an obvious one. Were we prepared for a pandemic? When "it" became a reality, were we ready? It is that question that shall be assessed first as we begin to try to understand the COVID-19 reality in the United States.

CHAPTER TWO

Preparing for a Pandemic: Were We Ready?

The world is ill-prepared to respond to a severe influenza pandemic or to any similarly global, sustained and threatening public health emergency.
—International Health Regulations Review Committee (2011)

There is no governing structure for a pandemic, and little more than vague political pressure to ensure limited access to life-sparing tools and medicines for more than half of the world's population.
—Laurie Garrett, Pulitzer Prize–winning science journalist

Introduction

It was the summer of 2005, and President George W. Bush was vacationing at his ranch in Crawford, Texas. His vacation reading included an advance copy of historian John M. Barry's newest book, *The Great Influenza*. He was quickly absorbed by what he was reading. In fact, he could not put it down. This book told the chilling tale of the 1918 Spanish flu pandemic. The impact of the book on the president would soon be apparent to all. When he returned to Washington, he called Fran Townsend (his top homeland security adviser) into the Oval Office. Giving her the galley of the forthcoming book, he said, "You've got to read this." Knowing that major pandemics happen every one hundred years or so and that U.S. public health experts were identifying a growing number of risks for novel disease outbreaks with the potential to ignite the next pandemic and having just read about the 1918 pandemic, the president made it clearly known what he felt needed to be done. In fact, he had a sense of great urgency about it. "We need a national strategy," he said.[1]

In 2005, public health experts in the United States and medical researchers across the globe were speaking of the growing evidence that the world was on the verge of a major pandemic outbreak. There was no certainty about which of the new virus strains being studied might mutate and be the cause of it, but there was no shortage of candidates. Of most immediate concern was an outbreak of a new avian influenza virus, the H5N1. In response to this new threat, President Bush initiated an ambitious national pandemic planning process that resulted in the development of a national strategy that was released on November 1, 2005. He spoke to the nation and warned, "A pandemic is a lot like a forest fire. If caught early it might be extinguished with limited damage. If allowed to smolder, undetected, it can grow into an inferno that can spread beyond our ability to control it."[2] As we shall see, a rather involved and impressive plan was laid out.[3] We shall also see that, despite the progress made by the Bush administration with respect to pandemic planning, support for this effort would wane over time, and our progress would be interrupted.

As President Barack Obama took office in 2009, he was soon greeted with a new influenza virus, the H1N1, which would become a minor pandemic before all was said and done. On April 22, 2009, to address the perceived H1N1 health threat, the Centers for Disease Control and Prevention (CDC) set up an emergency operations center. The CDC soon discovered that human-to-human H1N1 virus transmission, limited though it may be, was occurring in different countries around the world. The first press briefing took place shortly thereafter, but a national emergency was not declared until October 2, 2009. The H1N1 flu, a swine flu, had jumped to the human population. The roots of this virus were suspected to be in Southeast Asia, but the first known human cases were observed in Mexico. Between April 2009 and April 2010, the virus reached pandemic proportions. According to the CDC, there were 60.8 million H1N1 cases in the United States, with 12,469 deaths. This virus killed an estimated 203,000 people worldwide. Efforts to accelerate the production of a vaccine were undertaken. The first doses would become available in just twenty-six weeks.[4]

The H1N1 flu outbreak, while thankfully not as severe as some had originally feared, was nevertheless classified as a pandemic. The virus spread widely in April and May 2009, slowed through midsummer, and picked up again with a second wave in late summer as children returned to school. The peak came in late October and early November, and then it waned very quickly. A feared third wave never materialized. While the death rate was much lower than originally projected, the number of American cases, hospitalizations, and deaths were substantial enough to alert the Obama administration and public health experts that they needed to prepare for a more severe pandemic.[5] Despite the progress made during the Bush presidency starting in 2005, much more needed to be done. The Obama administration would prioritize pandemic preparedness anew.

By 2014, it was still very clear that the United States needed to do even more to be adequately prepared for a pandemic. President Obama proposed major new efforts, with major funding requests to Congress, to address the need as he perceived it. In the announcement advancing his proposals, the president explained his priorities: "If and when a new strain of flu, like the Spanish flu, crops up five years from now or a decade from now, we've made the investment and we're further along to be able to catch it. It's a smart investment for us to make." He also emphasized that "we're going to continue to have problems like this, particularly in a globalized world where you move from one side of the world to the other in a single day."[6] Despite a lack of Republican support in Congress, which would frustrate some of his legislative objectives to address this perceived threat, President Obama (like President Bush before him) prioritized pandemic preparedness.

An examination of American planning and preparedness efforts between the years 2005 and 2017 reveals many very positive steps forward, many interrupted steps, and too many steps not taken. As we turn to the task of summarizing these planning and preparedness activities, we need to keep several things in mind. Planning for a crisis, something everyone might support in the abstract, often loses out in the mix of more immediate concerns, resource limitations, and the politics of the moment. This inevitably makes the efforts to plan for the next crisis, however noble and well-intended, inconsistent and incomplete. Even with the wealth of information at their disposal and the consistent and excellent work of medical researchers and public health agencies to keep them informed, politicians are easily distracted from the coming crisis. Their attention and time are easily consumed by the minutia of the moment. The knowledge base and expertise necessary to be prepared for the crisis exists, but the willingness to engage is often distracted by the vagaries of partisan politics and the intense heat of the political moment. This is an unfortunate by-product of everyday politics in the United States.

Inconsistency and imperfection should not surprise us as we examine the path of our efforts to prepare for a global pandemic. On the other hand, it may not be unreasonable to suggest that on March 5, 2020, the president of the United States should have had some awareness of the efforts made by his two immediate predecessors to be prepared. Yet, as the first COVID-19 pandemic wave hit the United States, President Donald Trump asserted, "Nobody knew there would be a pandemic or epidemic of this proportion."

Pandemic Preparedness: 2005–2006

Most Americans have heard about the federal agency called the Centers for Disease Control and Prevention (CDC). However, they may not really know much about what the CDC actually does. The CDC began in the 1940s as a federal initiative to prevent the spread of malaria in the United States. Headquartered in Atlanta, Georgia, it began with a staff of only four hundred. Its original name was the Communicable Disease Center. In 1980, its official name was changed to the Centers for Disease Control and Prevention. Over the decades, the CDC has expanded the number of services it provides to the American public. Its primary mission is to protect American citizens from health and security threats nationally and internationally.

Today, the CDC employs over twelve thousand people. These CDC employees may be working within the United States or in more than 120 countries around the world. CDC researchers and scientists collaborate with researchers around the world to monitor the emergence of, and hopefully to contain the spread of, deadly new viruses and new disease threats. Among their number can be found epidemiologists, health scientists, health analysts, and research associates. In the 1950s, the work of the CDC was vital in efforts to control the spread of sexually transmitted diseases. In the 1960s, it led the efforts to address tuberculosis. In the 1980s, AIDS research became a new focus. The CDC has had numerous programs to address such things as chronic diseases, bioterrorism, and environmental health. It has proven to be instrumental in combating recent and serious health threats, such as the West Nile virus, the Zika virus, pandemic flu, and swine flu.

CDC research initiatives are constantly ongoing. All public health problems and potential problems are being studied and constantly analyzed, with the goal of protecting the public from new or looming health concerns. The CDC is responsible for maintaining an extensive database that includes recommendations and guidelines for the prevention of diseases. The research, expertise, and science-based recommendations of the CDC have guided American policy makers in addressing major public health concerns over the past seven decades. This would include the monitoring of and preparations for the possibility of a new epidemic or a pandemic.

By 2005, the CDC and health experts and researchers around the globe were in agreement that an influenza pandemic, the most serious one since the Spanish flu of 1918, was on the horizon. They were most concerned about a new virus that held the potential to pose a very great global health threat. This virus, the H5N1 flu strain (also known as the bird flu or avian influenza), held the potential to mutate into a deadly threat to humans should it become transmissible from human to human. The concerns over this new threat ignited a new and very serious round of pandemic preparedness around the world.[7]

Why did H5N1 cause such a global stir? Between 2003 and 2008, sixty-five countries had experienced animal (poultry) outbreaks of the H5N1 virus. In fact, the size of this outbreak was considered historic and unprecedented. In this same time period, fourteen countries had experienced confirmed human cases of H5N1. These human cases, 382 in number, had resulted in 241 deaths, for a death rate of 63 percent. Human-to-human transmission was thought to have already occurred in Indonesia. Indonesia had experienced the largest number of cases (133) and the highest death rate (81 percent).[8] The fatality rates cited in these initial cases were so high because the virus was binding to cells in the deep part of the lung. This meant that viral pneumonia was the first manifestation of the disease. But as the disease infected humans, it was likely that it would develop the capacity to bind to cells in the upper respiratory tract, much like seasonal influenzas do. As that happened, it was expected that the fatality rate would drop. Still, if it were to spread from human to human and reach pandemic proportions, it would have the potential to result in millions of deaths. Most of the cases reported in this early phase had been infected by direct contact with birds. The largest worldwide poultry outbreak ever recorded, combined with the spillover infections in humans, was of great concern. There was an even greater concern that should the virus mutate and become easily transmissible from human to human, a major pandemic would be inevitable.

By 2005, most scientific experts had been predicting that the next pandemic was on the horizon. In fact, they warned that the world was overdue for a major one. They were almost universal in their agreement that one would happen within the next ten to twenty years. A major pandemic could, many suggested, result in 5 million to 500 million deaths worldwide. The World Health Organization (WHO) more conservatively estimated 1.9 million to 7.5 million deaths. Fatality rates would obviously vary according to the resources that national health organizations had in place and the capacity of governments, guided by science, to respond in a timely and effective way. The H5N1 virus alerted all nations that a full-fledged pandemic disease that would spread around the globe, affecting entire nations at once, was a very real threat.[9] Most Americans were no doubt, and understandably, blissfully unaware of this perceived threat. But governments, including and especially the U.S. government, were very aware and were stirred to action.

Beginning in 2005, governmental planning for a possible pandemic animated government at all levels in the United States. The Department of Homeland Security (DHS), given the priorities of President Bush and the growing concerns in the scientific community about a global pandemic, developed a national strategy to guide the national, state, and local governments in preparing for an expected flu pandemic. The preparation would be based on the assumption that this global pandemic would be the worst one in one hundred years. This national strategy, once developed, called for the implementation of over three hundred actions by federal departments and agencies. It also articulated expectations for nonfederal entities (state and local governments, the private sector, critical infrastructure, individual citizens, etc.). The key responsibilities of the federal government would be coordinating the response of federal agencies, funding and supporting the development of vaccines and antivirals, stockpiling vaccines and other countermeasures, stockpiling essential equipment for first responders, providing national leadership to guide and (as necessary) support the state and local governments, and coordinating with other nations. State and local governments as well as private-sector actors were also to develop specific plans for their response to a pandemic.[10]

Warnings that a new pandemic might be something on the order of the 1918 Spanish flu intensified the concern among governments at all levels. The Spanish flu unfolded without warning. Even as it began to spread, our government and most governments around the world remained quiet and inactive. They were focused on World War I. Decisions were made to not alarm the public for fear of weakening morale and harming the war effort and the economy. The science of the era eventually, after having much tragic experience with the disease, began to speak with alarm of a new and deadly flu virus. Government leaders and the media initially persisted in the belief that it was just a typical flu bug and could be handled in the natural course of events. Even some medical journals opined in the early days of the crisis that the new flu was no more serious than any flu without the "new name."[11]

In the United States, the federal government made little mention of the pandemic and provided precious little leadership. President Woodrow Wilson had focused the nation on an all-out effort to prepare the nation for, and then to implement, its entrance into World War I. Nothing, including a pandemic, would be allowed to interfere with or dampen enthusiasm for that total effort. President Wilson never made one speech or issued any public statements about an influenza pandemic. The state and local governments were pretty much left on their own to deal with the greatest public health emergency that the nation had ever faced. The media, encouraged by the government to support the war effort and rally the nation, was willing and eager to do its patriotic part to win the war to end all wars. It more or less self-censored itself as the pandemic emerged and downplayed the seriousness of the disease. Perhaps they believed the disease was not all that serious. More likely, they did not want to report anything that would detract from or dampen support for the war effort.[12]

The Spanish flu did not even originate in Spain. There is strong circumstantial evidence to suggest that the first cases were in the United States (at a military base in Kansas). It is thought that some recruits from Haskell County, Kansas, carried the virus to Camp Funston. Within a few weeks, over one thousand recruits on the base were ill enough to require hospitalization. It is thought that soldiers from this camp brought the virus to other camps across the country as they were restationed from camp to camp. The cities surrounding these camps would be the first hot spots for an influenza outbreak in the United States. Even after seeing what was happening and being warned about its implications, the federal government did not stop reassigning soldiers from one camp to another. It is also thought that as American troops were transferred overseas, they took the virus with them. There had been flu outbreaks in Europe, but these would spike dramatically with the arrival of American troops. As this was happening, neither the American news media nor the media in any of the nations involved as combatants in the Great War provided anything resembling complete and accurate reporting. Spain, a neutral country during the war, was the first country to report openly and accurately about the evolving crisis, hence, the inaccurate label "Spanish flu."[13]

The Spanish flu came in three waves. Most epidemics and pandemics come in waves. The Spanish flu ultimately killed between 30 million and 50 million people worldwide, including 675,000 Americans. It infected 25 percent of the American population. The first wave was relatively mild. Two-thirds of the deaths occurred during the second wave. Three brutal months that began in the fall of 1918 were the deadliest time Americans had ever experienced in their history. Surprisingly, most flu victims were young and otherwise healthy adults. There were, of course, no effective drugs or vaccines to treat or prevent the spread of this killer flu. It would kill more people in less time than any disease before or since. American medical facilities were overwhelmed and stressed to the breaking point. As corpses piled up, citizens were ordered to wear masks, and schools, theaters, businesses, and many public places were shuttered altogether.[14] Needless to say, no one was prepared for the Spanish flu. Given the lessons one might hope were learned from that historic pandemic, it would be reasonable that warnings of a new pandemic of similar proportion would spur efforts to prepare for it. One would reasonably expect this to be a priority. Taking a closer look at the planning process that took place during the H5N1 scare reveals both the value and the limitations of pandemic preparedness.

As the federal government began planning and preparing federal departments and agencies for their roles in responding to a pandemic, DHS directed state and local communities to begin their planning. However, these state and local preparations revealed a lack of consensus about the best policies and strategies. Among business and private-sector actors, the effectiveness of planning efforts and the quality of relationships deemed necessary for the creation and implementation of pandemic plans remained questionable. During the planning period, a majority of global corporations had prepared and put in place reasonable flu pandemic plans, but a majority of small businesses would do very little, if any, planning.[15] This was of great concern inasmuch as small businesses would be among the most vulnerable during any pandemic outbreak. An even greater concern that emerged during the planning process was that businesses of all sizes reported an apparent lack of any coordination with the public sector. In 2006, 90 percent of all business entities surveyed indicated that they had not interacted with government at any level with respect to pandemic planning.[16]

Early warning is considered very critical with respect to containing the spread of an epidemic or pandemic. Seeing what is coming and acting to address it in a timely manner is essential. Waiting until it arrives and reacting to it is the beginning of failure. State and local governments were thus instructed to improve critical public health surveillance of both the human and animal populations. To the fullest extent possible, the H5N1 planning guidelines emphasized that the collaboration of public health, the medical community, agriculture, and business must be enhanced to promote improved surveillance of the human and animal populations for signs of disease. Ideally, this would be a part of an early-warning system.[17]

Public health surveillance of the human population requires a systematic collection and interpretation of data. A global pandemic requires an integrated worldwide network that brings health practitioners, researchers, and governments together across national boundaries. State and local communities both need the guidance of national entities, such as the CDC and the National Institutes of Health (NIH), and international entities, such as the World Health Organization (WHO), as valuable sources of information. Public health surveillance is one of the most important weapons to be enhanced in the effort to avert the most severe impacts of epidemics and pandemics. The improvement of health surveillance capacities was thus one of the major objectives of the H5N1 planning process at all levels.[18]

The H5N1 planning process emphasized that vaccination was the most reliable way to limit the impact of a pandemic. It is the responsibility of the federal government and the drug industry to collaborate on a vaccination plan and to implement it as quickly as possible. Local governments would, however, be critically involved in the distribution process. Local H5N1 plans were to include the designation of public treatment centers and points of vaccine distribution. But, suffice it to say, a pandemic would emerge and engulf the nation before any vaccine was available. Even an effort to begin working in advance on a vaccine for a specific virus, such as the H5N1, would not necessarily make a vaccine available before a pandemic unfolds. The mutation of the virus that will cause the pandemic cannot be predicted or known until it happens—when the pandemic wave begins. Under the best of circumstances, once a pandemic wave commences, it can take a year to eighteen months to produce an effective vaccine. It can take even years longer in some cases.

It can be said that the federal government's role in vaccine development is perhaps its most important job. The pharmaceutical industry is a trillion-dollar enterprise, but vaccines make up only 3 percent of the market.[19] The industry does a reasonable job with seasonal flu vaccines, but it must be remembered that influenza viruses constantly mutate. This means that each year, as new mutations occur, new versions of seasonal vaccines must be developed. This process takes many months. It can take years of research and testing and over a billion dollars to develop a new vaccine. Because the drug companies find it too costly and unprofitable to make and store pandemic vaccines, they are largely dependent on federal funding for research, development, and manufacturing. The same applies for many countermeasures needed to respond to a pandemic. Without federal funding, the private sector simply is not incentivized to meet the need.[20] Thus, a public-private partnership under the Biomedical Advanced

Research and Development Authority's (BARDA) pan flu program contracts with the private sector to develop pan flu countermeasures.

In their 2005–2006 planning for a pandemic, most state and local governments followed the advice of the WHO that available medications and what was expected to be a limited supply of any new vaccine that may be developed first be given to essential personnel as they became available.[21] Essential personnel included, in most plans, medical personnel. Also included were public health workers, emergency responders, police, firefighters, and critical infrastructure personnel. Many also included workers in the transportation industry responsible for the delivery of foods and medicines. Other nations developed similar lists of essential personnel for vaccine distribution.[22] Even with this planning, it was still probable that the shortages of treatment options and the lack of a vaccine at the beginning of a pandemic outbreak would leave the public in a precarious position without sufficient protection. This led to an emphasis on what might be called defensive strategies. These strategies would place great responsibilities and demands on government at all levels.

The expected shortages of countermeasures, the absence of a vaccine, and the inevitable overcrowding of hospitals in a pandemic crisis meant that pandemic planners were expected to be prepared to identify and efficiently implement necessary defensive measures as a pandemic threat level emerged. These defensive measures include things like social distancing, respiratory measures, and various hygiene measures. It was also seen as inevitable that school closings, bans on public gathering, travel bans, business closures, and even quarantine would be needed to slow the course of a pandemic. The planning needed to include triggering mechanisms for these defensive measures to ensure that they could be implemented in the most timely and effective way.[23]

In reality, it was understood that many states and communities would struggle to implement these measures in the most advantageous and timely way. A community might well be in the midst of a pandemic wave before these sorts of measures were implemented. The tardiness of some to implement would no doubt mean that the measures would need to be even more restrictive when implemented. This would not keep the disease and its impacts from becoming more severe than it might otherwise have been with an earlier and more efficient implementation, but it would flatten the curve, or the spread, of the disease. This would take some of the pressure off overburdened hospitals.

Given the expected shortages of medical interventions and the absence of a vaccine at the outset of a pandemic, it followed that most individuals and families would have to arrange for their own safety. This meant that risk communication and public education would be an important part of pandemic planning. Communicating the risks of a pandemic and educating the public about important and necessary self-defense measures to mitigate these risks was another critical emphasis of the H5N1 planning process. Suffice it to say, this would be a difficult challenge that government at all levels would need to manage in any crisis situation.

Crises come in many shapes and forms. They may come in the form of man-made accidents, natural disasters, or public health epidemics, to name just a few. Each major crisis will bear directly on the lives and well-being of citizens and societies. Among the most important components in governmental planning to address a crisis is a strategy for timely, accurate, and effective communication. This includes interagency and intergovernmental communication and, of critical importance in a pandemic scenario, the communication of political leaders (the president, governors, mayors, etc.) to the public. Political leaders must understand the truth of the crisis situation. They must know how to implement the plan and how to convey it to the public. They must provide accurate and timely information to the public and to all governmental actors. They must provide, in part through effective communication strategies, the leadership needed to guide the public through all stages of the crisis.[24]

Communicating the risks associated with a possible H5N1 pandemic (or any pandemic) was another important focus of the H5N1 planning process. It was essential to educate the public about what a pandemic would mean to them and how they should incorporate that meaning into their lives. They especially needed to know about and be instructed on the appropriate and necessary self-defense measures they would need to take to mitigate the risks to themselves, their families, and to society at large. A pandemic is not something that most Americans have on their radar screens. In fact, public surveys in 2005–2006 showed that many employers did not believe that a public health emergency would ever impact their businesses. They also showed that most Americans would not be prepared for a severe public health emergency.[25] This made educating and informing the public even more important as a priority. Social scientists have been studying and analyzing people's responses to risk communication for decades. The possibility for a sound pandemic risk communication and public education strategy existed to be sure, but it was (and would remain) largely undeveloped.[26]

The communication of risk and public education is complex. Done well, it requires coordination among various types of experts, including subject-matter experts, risk and decision analysts to identify information critical to the decisions of various audiences, psychologists to design

messages and evaluate their success, and communication systems special-
ists to ensure that tested messages get communicated within the crisis
response system.[27] There is no foolproof system for doing any of this, but
the work to design and implement more effective strategies is ongoing.
The best communication strategies will still be imperfect. Even with the
best plans, communication breakdowns and failures are an all too common feature in emergency response activities. The same can be said for
planning in general.

In 2009, as the H1N1 pandemic struck, the United States and most
nations had reasonable pandemic plans in place. These plans included
excellent recommendations and outlined the critical steps to be taken.
But, as we often find out with tragic consequences, plans do not equal
preparation. Too many world leaders ignored the plans or were simply too
slow to act. Simply put, they failed to do their job. Fortunately, this pandemic was not particularly severe, but it did alert us to an important variable to be considered. Plans may be imperfect, but one of the major
reasons for their failure is the human element. The failure of leadership is
often the most devastating and tragic failure of all.

One final concern that came to the fore during the H5N1 planning
process, although not dealt with in any detail in the federal, state, and
local plans that were produced, was the ethical dimension of a pandemic
threat. Planners recognized that the allocation of scarce resources, including medical supplies and vaccines when they became available, gave rise
to ethical questions. The same was said to be true with respect to the
application of social distancing and other control measures as they relate
to concerns about civil liberties. One study did a content analysis of local
pandemic plans and found a striking lack of ethical analysis and direction.[28] This should be a concern. Why? Because when a pandemic strikes
and spreads quickly across the nation, there would be very little time, if
any, to reflect on ethical concerns. It would be impossible to adjust public
health, medical, and response systems on the run to enable them to make
ethical decisions. Serious ethical concerns such as those associated with
the allocation of scarce resources or the constraints on civil liberties that
may be imposed cannot be reasonably addressed in the middle of an
unfolding crisis. They need much advance consideration and planning.
This suggests the necessity, or at least the utility, of including trained ethi-
cists in the pandemic planning process.

As the United States completed its pandemic planning in the shadow
of the H5N1 threat, designing that "national strategy" that President Bush
had said was needed, very good progress was made. However, there
remained obvious concerns that needed to be revisited, and the planning

process would ideally have to be an ongoing process. It would also be necessary to properly fund pandemic response capacities. Indeed, from 2006 to 2013, federal funding for pandemic response was enhanced. The U.S. Congress allocated $5.6 billion to implement the first two years of the pandemic plan just produced. When the 2009 H1N1 strain broke out, an emergency supplemental appropriation of $6.1 billion was allocated. But, over time, the willingness of the Congress to invest the necessary dollars for pandemic preparedness rapidly declined. By 2014, BARDA's pan-flu plan had seen its budget reduced to the point that the Department of Health and Human Services (HHS) concluded that BARDA would not be able to award the new contracts required for maintaining the existing stockpiles of pandemic countermeasures. The HHS reported in 2015 that given the reduced allocations for preparedness, it would be impossible to mount an efficient and effective pandemic response.[29]

Pandemic Preparedness: 2009–2017

In his economic stimulus package submitted to Congress in 2009, President Barack Obama proposed new funding for pandemic prepared-ness. However, Congress eliminated the $870 million slated for this purpose. Understandably perhaps, cutting funding for flu pandemic pre-paredness was easily targeted in the context of the economic crisis that was facing the nation in the aftermath of the 2008 crash of the housing market. Many members of Congress, especially Republican members, expressed the notion that spending for pandemic preparedness seemed to be a luxury that was not affordable. Even in the best of times, spending money to address a crisis that scientists tell us might occur at some impre-cisely defined future time is a tough sell in the political universe. As Congress was cutting proposed funding for pandemic preparedness, that imprecisely defined future became all too immediate.

The H1N1 flu, another new virus, was breaking out. It would eventu-ally be classified as a pandemic. As noted earlier, it was thankfully not as severe as originally feared. But this pandemic did kill an estimated 203,000 people worldwide, including over 12,000 Americans. Over 60 million American cases would be recorded. Early in the H1N1 pandemic, when the first wave hit in April and May 2009, there was no vaccine available. But studies did show that most Americans were quick to adopt two recommended defensive strategies. In the first weeks, almost two-thirds of Americans said that they and members of their family had begun to wash their hands or clean them with sanitizer more frequently. Most also made preparations to stay at home if they or a family member got sick. Four in ten Americans noted that they took great care to avoid exposure to people who were displaying any flu-like symptoms.[30]

A majority of Americans reported that they had followed media reports on the progress in H1N1 vaccine development. A vaccine was produced in just twenty-six weeks, an unexpectedly rapid time frame. To its credit, the federal government had expedited this work. But initial reports that the vaccine might not be as effective or as safe as originally thought and the failure to produce it in a timely manner and in quantities necessary to be widely available discouraged many Americans from feeling comfortable with it. Fears about the safety of the new vaccine caused many to be reluctant and unwilling to expose themselves to it. The lack of public confidence in the vaccine and the bottlenecks in vaccine development that slowed the process for getting the new vaccine to the marketplace were major problems. In a more severe and deadly pandemic, these issues would have increased the death toll significantly.[31]

The H1N1 pandemic prompted a massive and coordinated response from the U.S. public health system. As such, it provided the first opportunity to implement state and federal pandemic plans that had been produced in response to the H5N1 scare a few years earlier. While the combined responses of government at all levels were generally commendable, the policies and plans developed did not adequately address many of the specific events and circumstances that unfolded during the H1N1 outbreak. The Association of State and Territorial Health Officials (ASTHO) prepared a report for the CDC assessing the national response to H1N1. Several deficiencies were noted, and recommendations were made to improve the public health response.[32]

The first item identified in the ASTHO report was the need for a more consistent, effective, and unified command structure. This would have benefited the response at all levels of government. The need for more timely guidance from the federal government was especially noted as well as the need for a more centralized approach to pandemic response to guide states and localities. Several additional items were identified for needed improvements. Delays in vaccine production and conflicting messages about its availability caused considerable confusion for the public. It also damaged the credibility of government at all levels. Better consistency and improved efforts were needed nationally with respect to disease surveillance strategies, data collection, and analysis. Federal stockpiling measures needed to be improved to better assist state and local response activities that were influenced by the supply chain of critical medical countermeasures. There were too many delays and conflicts in federal guidelines on respiratory protection. This led to confusion and shortages in supplies and delayed the release of state and local stockpiles. The H1N1 pandemic strained public health laboratory capacity at both the federal and state levels. Finally, CDC communication efforts were successful with a range of audiences, but they fell far short of reaching and meeting the needs of vulnerable populations and minority communities.[33] It was generally agreed that prior pandemic planning had been helpful in responding to the H1N1 outbreak, but it did not prove to be sufficient to meet all the challenges the pandemic would pose. It was also clear that improvements would be needed before the United States could be said to be ready for a more severe and lethal pandemic.

The H1N1 pandemic came at a vulnerable time for cash-strapped state and local public health departments. It broke out just as the U.S. Congress had reduced the money slated for flu preparedness in the 2009 economic stimulus package. Even under the best of conditions, the government does not spend money in a way that makes preparing for future pandemics a priority. This is not to say that Congress does not allocate funds to address public health concerns. It is to say that the money typically gets spent in a reaction to public health emergencies and not usually in anticipation of them. The funding is easier to come by on a disease-by-disease basis and usually *after* a crisis has already begun. During the 2013–2016 Ebola crisis, Congress did appropriate over $5 billion to address the health emergency. This funding came about five months after international health groups had identified it as an urgent crisis.[34] That sort of reactive approach, a delay in responding, simply is not helpful in a pandemic scenario. The Ebola epidemic would demonstrate just how ill prepared the United States was for a major public health crisis.

Ebola (Ebola hemorrhagic fever) is a rare and deadly disease caused by infection with one of the four Ebola virus species known to cause disease in humans. It was first discovered in 1976 near the Ebola River in what is now the Democratic Republic of the Congo. Since 1976, outbreaks have occurred sporadically in Africa. As the new outbreak took flight in 2013, the United States and the world were much too slow to react. Why should the United States react? All advanced nations know the need to address epidemic outbreaks in developing countries is essential to prevent the global spread of diseases and to assist nations where the health systems are inadequate to the challenge. In other words, it is not only for humanitarian reasons that the United States and other countries respond to epidemics in the underdeveloped countries of the world. They do it to protect the health of their citizens as well by containing and preventing the spread of disease.

As the new outbreak of Ebola began in 2009, the United States had just made cuts in the funding of essential public health agencies that would be needed to respond to any global medical emergency. It can be said that the United States fumbled its response to the Ebola epidemic before it even began, neglecting experiments to make vaccines and drugs against the virus and cutting critical funding to key public health agencies. But the United States was not alone in its failures.

The worldwide response to the new Ebola outbreak in West Africa was too slow. The WHO admitted as much and said that it had come up short with respect to the resources needed to respond. The epidemic began to spread quickly, and it overwhelmed the fragile health care systems of poor West African nations. It killed thousands of people. The monthslong delay by developed countries in providing the resources necessary to respond to the outbreak meant many more would die. In addition to the tragic consequences for West Africans, the world's slowness to respond to the Ebola crisis highlighted major inadequacies in the world's ability to respond to global public health emergencies. Every nation would have to rethink its preparations for a major global public health crisis. The U.S. government knew that it had significant work to do to address this concern, but before it could begin to act, another crisis was at its doorstep.

From May 2015 through December 2016, an outbreak of the Zika virus presented a new medical threat to the United States. The Zika virus, a flavivirus that is primarily transmitted by *Aedes* mosquitoes, had rapidly spread throughout the Americas beginning in May 2015. A Zika virus infection during pregnancy is known to be the cause of microcephaly and other congenital abnormalities, and infection is also associated with neurologic disorders.[35] By the spring of 2016, there were almost twenty-seven hundred travel-related cases of Zika in the United States. Things were much worse in U.S. territories, where more than fourteen thousand locally acquired cases had been reported. As this new crisis began to unfold, Congress had yet to pass a funding bill. This presented the Obama administration with the difficult challenge of having to initiate a response without new resources. The administration decided to redirect money earmarked for other purposes, including the Ebola response, to support Zika research and response efforts. Virtually every public health expert agreed that the response to the Zika crisis, like the response to Ebola, was weakened by a fragmented and partisan U.S. political system that was simply too slow and inadequate in the face of an emergency.[36]

In early February 2016, President Obama had sent a proposal to Congress requesting $1.9 billion in supplemental funding to strengthen local public health responses to the Zika threat. This included funding for hard-hit U.S. territories. Other major priorities considered critical included expanded Zika testing in the United States and support for research on a new vaccine. In addition to these priorities, given the global nature of the Zika threat, $400 million was earmarked for providing assistance abroad. Both the House and the Senate countered with alternative bills. The House bill authorized only one-third of the amount requested by the president. The Senate bill opted for the reallocation of existing Ebola funding to address the Zika response. With a congressional deadlock and no legislation forthcoming, President Obama had no choice but to use his administrative authority to move $81 million already allocated for biomedical research, Ebola, and other health programs to keep a Zika vaccine study going and to support local governments.[37] Every dollar that was spent from the spring through the fall of 2016 on the Zika outbreak, a period regarded as time sensitive and critical for responding to the Zika threat, was money that the administration had had to reallocate from other uses. This money would not be enough, and it would soon run out.

As the fall of 2016 arrived, public health experts called the American response to Zika insufficient. This was polite. The shifting of money away from existing public health initiatives, including Ebola response and prevention, undermined national and local efforts to prevent other disease outbreaks. In October 2016, Congress finally acted. It finally allocated $1.1 billion to combat the threat posed by the Zika virus. Still, a portion of this funding was taken from the Ebola response. Though they were happy to finally see the new funding, public health officials continued to vent their frustration that Congress had taken so long to act. By October, the virus had spread to twenty-five thousand people in the United States and its territories. Experts warned that such a delayed response in a serious pandemic scenario would most certainly result in a tragic increase in the death toll.[38]

The fact is that even if we have developed good plans for responding to an epidemic or a pandemic, this does not automatically translate into maintained preparedness and a successful response. Even without new disease outbreaks and tardy legislative responses, plans do not translate into the actions necessary to be prepared. Following its pandemic planning in 2005–2006, the Department of Homeland Security (DHS) did a follow-up study of pandemic preparedness in 2014. The DHS Office of Inspector General issued a report that concluded that the DHS had not effectively managed pandemic personal protective equipment (PPE) and antiviral countermeasures. DHS had not conducted a needs assessment with regard to purchasing pandemic preparedness supplies, and it had not managed its stockpile of PPE and medical countermeasures. It had not developed and implemented stockpile replacement plans, executed adequate contract oversight processes, or ensured compliance with departmental guidelines.[39] In short, there was no assurance that DHS would be prepared for a pandemic.

As the experiences of the H1N1, Ebola, and Zika outbreaks left their mark in relatively short order amid growing concerns among public health experts and researchers about a more serious crisis on the horizon, there was a growing and uncomfortable awareness that the threat of a global pandemic was heating up and that the U.S. government was still not adequately prepared to deal with it. General Mark Welsh, U.S. Air Force chief of staff from 2012 to 2016, had overseen the military's contributions in response to the Ebola and Zika outbreaks and was among those who were quite worried about American preparedness. During the Ebola and Zika episodes, Welsh observed what he called a lack of planning and effective leadership. He concluded that his observations gave him great doubts about the U.S. government's ability to respond to a global medical crisis. He worried that the United States simply could not be expected to overcome a lack of persistent planning or to deploy experts and support staff to affected areas in an effective manner so as to contain and mitigate the spread of a deadly virus. Despite all the planning already done, much of it very sound, we simply were not yet adequately prepared.[40] This was not only an American concern but also a global concern.

Victor Dzau, president of the U.S. National Academy of Medicine, speaking from the 2016 World Health Summit in Berlin, Germany, reported on the findings of an international study that the academy had been asked to implement for the CDC. The academy, in consultation with hundreds of experts around the world, examined then current disease response preparedness activities and projected future response capacities. The report noted failures at all levels: "At the international level, there is a lack of coordination and resources; at the national level, there is a lack of public health infrastructure, capacity, and workforce; and at the local level, there is a lack of community trust and engagement."[41] The report concluded that the world was simply not prepared for a pandemic.

Several important lessons were clear to many American decision makers. The scattershot way the United States has typically dealt with its response to disease outbreaks is, given the nature of the threat, irrational. In fact, it often makes a bad situation worse. Its recent experiences indicated that the United States needed more sustained funding and persistent upgrades in planning and preparedness that would extend over many years. It was clear that the United States had worked to do some serious pandemic planning. But it was equally clear that if efforts to contain an outbreak at its source were to fail, the resources of the federal government would not be sufficient to prevent or control the spread of a pandemic across the nation. Equally concerning, the capacity of our leaders and policy makers to respond quickly, effectively, and intelligently to a fast-moving pandemic wave was unproven, perhaps even doubtful. None of these conclusions is particularly surprising. Efforts to address these concerns, and others like them, have kept presidents awake at night and made them determined to improve the nation's readiness. Like his predecessor, President Obama felt it was absolutely essential to keep the planning process in motion.

In the summer of 2009, in anticipation of the coming H1N1 outbreak, the recently inaugurated Obama gave the President's Council of Advisors on Science and Technology (PCAST) its first assignment. The president had noted that he was committed to integrating science into his day-to-day decisions. One of the primary decisions where science would be the most important variable was how to respond to the outbreak of a global pandemic. He wanted to know what a president needs to do to be prepared for an influenza pandemic. On August 7, 2009, PCAST met with the president and gave him its answer. Their response included the recommendation that a top-level White House official be devoted to planning for and responding to infectious disease threats. Over the course of his presidency, Obama pursued the goal of putting a pandemic infrastructure into place. This would culminate in the creation of a document titled the *Playbook for Early Response to High-Consequence Emerging Infectious Disease Threats and Biological Incidents*. This playbook was prepared to guide the work of responding to a public health emergency.[42]

Even before giving PCAST its first assignment, President Obama had made clear that his administration would have a commitment to science. In April 2009, speaking before the National Academy of Sciences, he said with some emphasis that "science is more essential for our prosperity, our security, our health, our environment, and our quality of life than it has ever been before." This was on April 27, just a few days after the CDC had set up an operations center and made its first public statement about the emerging H1N1 crisis.[43] It is clear that preparing for a pandemic was an Obama administration priority from day one, and it was a process that would be ongoing throughout the next eight years.

The rapid succession of global health episodes (H1N1, Ebola, Zika) would present both challenges that indicated pandemic planning was incomplete and opportunities to improve it. Perhaps one of the most frightening aspects of pandemic response is that so many decisions must be made rapidly, in a timely manner, and often based on limited data. PCAST recommended that one person be designated, preferably the homeland security adviser, to coordinate all pandemic policy development and to report directly to the president. Obama took this advice, and John Brennan, the assistant to the president for homeland security, was appointed to this task. He also established the White House National Security Council Directorate for Global Health Security and Biodefense. Among its most urgent tasks would be to prepare for future pandemics. By 2016, the work begun in 2009, combined with the experiences of the previous seven years, culminated in the production of the already mentioned pandemic playbook.

The *Playbook for Early Response to High-Consequence Emerging Infectious Disease Threats and Biological Incidents* was a sixty-nine-page document produced by the planning group in the president's National Security Council (NSC) and was designed to coordinate a response to an emerging disease threat anywhere in the world. It detailed decision-making rubrics to guide key decisions in what was hoped would be the most timely and efficient manner. Each section of the playbook included the specific questions that should be raised and the decisions that should be made at all levels within the national security apparatus. Perhaps worth noting here, officials were advised to question the numbers on viral spread, ensure appropriate diagnostic capacity, and make sure that the U.S. stockpiles of emergency resources were adequate and that their distribution would be efficient. The first question to be asked as a pandemic emerged, according to the playbook, was whether there was sufficient PPE for the health care workers who were to provide medical care. If supplies were deemed adequate, what are the triggers that signal the exhaustion of supplies? Are additional supplies available? If no, does this trigger the release of PPE from the Strategic National Stockpile to the states? Literally hundreds of questions, strategies, tactics, and triggers for policy decisions were laid out in the playbook. Every aspect of pandemic response, including the more dramatic decisions pertaining to such things as travel bans, social distancing protocols, school and business closures, quarantines, vaccine production, and economic impacts were covered.[44]

The playbook emphasized it was the responsibility of the White House to contain the risks of a potential pandemic. The stated objectives of the playbook made it abundantly clear that the national government would aggressively take the lead during a public health crisis: "The U.S. government will use all powers at its disposal to prevent, slow or mitigate the spread of an emerging infectious disease threat." The playbook offers as a central premise that "the American public will look to the U.S. government for action when multi-state or other significant events occur."[45] The plan stressed that it was critically important that the federal response be prepared to present a "unified message" to manage the American public's questions and concerns during a crisis. "Early coordination of risk communication through a single federal spokesperson is critical," the playbook urges.[46] This playbook created for NSC staff was intended to help federal officials confront a wide range of potential biological threats. But it was undoubtedly the building concerns over a potential global pandemic that had been raised by science and made more relevant as an urgent concern by the events of recent years that was the primary motivation for the playbook.

It should be noted that the NSC playbook was not by any means complete. Some of the specific decisions to be anticipated in a pandemic scenario needed to be fleshed out in greater detail, and some important items were sparsely discussed. It must be noted that the playbook was seen as a part of a process set in motion with the 2005–2006 planning during the H5N1 scare; however, out of necessity, this process would have to continue, and the planning would be ongoing. It is said that when General Eisenhower was planning for D-Day, the first thing he did when he had planned out was to plan it again. He supposedly said, "Plans are nothing; planning is everything." Given the unforeseen twists a new virus may take, the unique characteristics of each public health crisis, and the inconsistency of follow-through inherent with respect to most plans, it can certainly be said of pandemic preparedness that plans are nothing, but planning is everything. It should thus be no surprise that as he left office, President Obama emphasized the need to continue the planning and preparedness efforts for the next pandemic.

Conclusion: Passing the Torch

The transition of the American presidency from one administration to the next is an intricate and important dance to be performed. The outgoing administration, especially if it has served two terms and knows that its end date is certain, has prepared extensive briefings for the incoming administration. Transition officials and appointees of the new administration literally show up the day after the election eager to receive briefings and in-depth briefing books from their predecessors. Even when there is a major philosophical difference and significant policy differences between the two administrations, it is critical for the incoming team to understand the ongoing work in the departments and agencies they will soon head. They need to be thoroughly versed on the significant items, especially the major challenges, that will require their immediate attention. The experience and knowledge of the outgoing team can be an indispensable asset to an incoming administration as it sets about the task of hitting the ground with its feet moving, so to speak. The Obama administration and its department and agency leaders had prepared its detailed transition briefings for many months. President Obama had been very impressed with the detailed and helpful briefings the outgoing Bush administration had provided for his new team. He was determined that his administration prepare for an equally impressive hand off to his successor.

The 2016 election happened. Then nothing happed. Obama administration departments and agencies waited for the representatives of the new administration of Donald Trump to appear. Across all departments and agencies, a similar story played itself out. Trump appointees were few and far between. Those few that did show up were shockingly uninformed about the functions of their new workplace. They were, in many instances, not very much interested in the briefings. Some even threw away the briefing books that had been prepared for them. This transition, documented by Michael Lewis in his book *The Fifth Risk*, was unlike any seen in contemporary times. While there would remain within the U.S. civil service those career professionals whose knowledge, dedication, and proactivity would keep the machinery running, one had to wonder whether the incoming political appointees who would head their departments and agencies might throw more than a few wrenches into that machinery.[47]

This concern was not political or ideological but one of simple logic. What damage might unintentionally be done by political appointees not interested in or hostile to the professionals whose experience and knowledge could be useful to their objectives and absolutely essential to keep the ship of state afloat? Politics and policy aside, one could be forgiven for wondering how much damage might be done by an uninformed, short-sighted administration not interested in the details of governing. To be fair, one must also readily admit that damage can also be done by an administration that is more informed and farsighted.

The Trump administration was thoroughly briefed on the NSC pandemic playbook. They were told to expect a potential pandemic and to continue the efforts to better prepare for one. A tabletop exercise was prepared and presented to Trump's incoming team. It was a sober briefing as the incoming team was walked through a scenario for the worst pandemic since 1918. Media reports that circulated in the spring of 2020 suggested that the Trump team was little interested in the briefing. Indeed, and as shall be discussed in our assessment of the American response to the COVID-19 pandemic, the playbook seemed to have been shelved and forgotten early on in the Trump administration.

At the beginning of 2017 and the start of a new administration in the White House, a new avian influenza strain emerged and reanimated concerns about a possible influenza pandemic. The H7N9 virus had spread across China. It had mostly infected poultry, but it had begun to spread from chickens to humans. Almost nine out of ten humans infected with H7N9 came down with pneumonia. Seventy-five percent of the infected humans experienced severe respiratory problems and ended up in intensive care. Forty-one percent of infected humans died. Once again, experts were warning of a possible pandemic. The H7N9 was China's fifth and largest outbreak of avian influenza. According to the experts, at the beginning of 2017, this was the influenza strain with the greatest potential to cause the next global influenza pandemic.[48] Most Americans undoubtedly paid little attention to this news. There was little evidence that the new administration did either.

As 2017 began with the news of a heightened risk of a global pandemic, the Trump administration had not yet appointed senior officials to head the key federal agencies responsible for pandemic preparedness or responding to a public health emergency. There were leadership vacancies in the Department of Health and Human Services (HHS), the National Institutes of Health (NIH), and the Centers for Disease Control and Prevention (CDC). In addition to leadership vacancies, these agencies were targeted for significant budget cuts under the proposed Trump budget for 2018.[49] Congress would ultimately not support all the cuts, but clearly the new administration did not prioritize public health concerns in its budgetary decisions. In fact, that original proposal had called for an 18 percent reduction (about $5.8 billion) in the NIH biomedical research funding that would play an essential role in equipping the federal government to detect new disease outbreaks and vaccine production. It would have also compromised international health research efforts and negatively impacted efforts to contain any outbreak that might occur.[50] The fact is that the appointment of leadership in these agencies that are responsible for the nation's health security and providing the funding resources needed to ensure that they can effectively produce vaccines, implement defensive measures to control disease outbreaks, and provide national leadership in a public health crisis should have been a top priority at the beginning of 2017.

Even before 2017, and despite the progress made in the two previous administrations to address pandemic preparedness, there was a growing concern within the scientific community that the U.S. government needed to strengthen its commitment to pandemic preparedness. Even though the Bush and the Obama administrations had made progress toward this goal, as 2017 began, there was considerable worry that too much still needed to be done before we could consider ourselves prepared for a major global pandemic. The needs they stressed were based on both the science of the matter and the lessons learned from the experiences accumulated over the previous years with disease outbreaks, including and especially the H1N1 pandemic and the Ebola and Zika outbreaks. The plans that had been produced needed to be improved. Once again, the truth of General Eisenhower's old adage ("Plans are nothing; planning is everything") had been borne out.

The needs that were articulated at the beginning of 2017 were based on the experience and knowledge gained by the previous two administrations. As has been shown in the summary of these experiences in this chapter, there were obvious and straightforward items to be pursued as the planning process continued. It was essential to ensure that national leadership during any national health crisis be upgraded and prioritized. The federal government needed to present a "unified message" to guide state and local officials and manage the American public's questions and concerns during a crisis. This meant refining the work of the NSC planning body and the appointment of a lead person to be the source of all federal statements and advisories during a public health emergency. This also included the coordination of all federal agencies to interact smoothly and efficiently during an unfolding crisis. It meant making sure that public health agencies, especially the CDC, provided scientifically sound directives to guide the actions of state and local first responders. This needed to be done in a timely and coordinated fashion and with detail, clarity and a unified message. It meant informing the public with a consistent and science-based strategy. Improving public awareness with accurate and timely information was said to be a priority of the utmost importance. This federal "leadership" need was based on the understanding that while a multistate effort would be needed in response to a pandemic, this effort needed to have direction, and it needed to be consistent from state to state. States and citizens alike would be best served by a well-organized federal effort to inform and guide all actors, public and private.

The other needs to be met were also very obvious. These included more consistent support for the research and development of vaccines, therapeutics, and diagnostics. It was of critical importance to invest the resources and the effort required to replenish the stockpiles of countermeasure and response supplies that first responders would need during a public health emergency. It was important that the federal government be prepared to be aggressively active in assisting the states and localities as their systems became overwhelmed and their supplies came up short.

On the international level, it was regarded as essential for the United States to continue and enhance its coordination with other nations in ongoing research and to improve the coordination of global response activities. Each of these needs would require sustained and persistent work to ensure that the United States was prepared for a global health crisis such as a pandemic.

Any objective assessment of infectious disease outbreaks in the decade preceding the passing of the torch to a new administration in 2017 made it clear that the United States and the world needed to recognize that they were not nearly as prepared as they needed to be for a global health crisis. All informed sources told us that the world needed to be better prepared through enhanced coordination, more investment, more research, improved systems for disease surveillance, and better infrastructure. Any minimal attention to and understanding of what the public health community and the scientific research were telling the world in January 2017 would have caused any new administration—or any reasonable person for that matter—to acknowledge that continuing and enhancing the work of pandemic preparedness was an important national priority.

Presidents Bush and Obama, one Republican and the other Democrat, had both recognized this priority and acted on it. They knew (as should we all) that a pandemic is not political. A virus is not a Republican or a Democrat; it is a hungry beast looking for its next meal. During a pandemic, humanity is a tasty steak that the virus will efficiently devour if given the chance. When it shows up at the table ready to dine, it is too late. With no immunity to the new disease, human beings are already cooked and ready to be served up. Pandemics are not really something to react to when they show up. Pandemics are something to prepare for well before they arrive. As this was well understood by his two predecessors, one can be sure that this message was relayed to President Trump and his incoming team in January 2017.

Before we begin to analyze exactly what the Trump administration did or did not do with the message relayed to it during the transition, it is important to understand elements in the American cultural and political environments that would exert a very important influence on the course of American pandemic planning between 2017 and 2020 as well as the national response to COVID-19. These influences would often, or so it would seem, have a greater impact than science on the decisions made and the actions taken as the worst pandemic in one hundred years showed up for its dinner.

CHAPTER THREE

Politics, Science, and Partisan Warfare

There are two things, science and opinion; the former begets knowledge, the latter ignorance.

—Hippocrates

The saddest aspect of life right now is that science gathers knowledge faster than society gathers wisdom.

—Isaac Asimov

Introduction

We have all heard the expression that there are no atheists in foxholes. The suggestion is that in the face of death on the battlefield, we will reach out to God, even if we were not predisposed to do so previously. In this same vein, when we are sick, most of us reach out to science and medicine for salvation. Most people would probably agree that in the midst of the COVID-19 pandemic, rejecting scientific consensus in favor of anti-science beliefs or preferences would have been a deadly mistake. One would hope that the prevailing attitude during any public health crisis would be to trust science and let the science lead. Yet, human history, including recent American history, shows us that science is easily rejected or denied when its findings offend or threaten the vested interests of the powers that be. Ideology and rhetoric are all too commonly employed to contradict or discredit the evidence that science may produce. It is also quite apparent to even the casual observer that much of what humans do, especially in the public policy arena, is done in willful denial of facts.

Science is not political, or so every scientist will insist. Yet, every statement of a scientifically observable fact may be of political significance insofar as it either supports or challenges the prevailing values of the existing culture and the existing power structure. The political consumers of scientific discoveries are typically more interested in a narrative that defines reality as their ideological and political interests or preferences prefer or dictate. The facts are accepted, massaged, manipulated, or denied as their interests and their struggle to attain or enhance their power may require. This is precisely why the Catholic Church accused Galileo of heresy.

In April 1633, the Catholic Church began its inquisition of Galileo Galilei. Galileo was a physicist, astronomer, and one of the greatest scientists of his era. He was put on trial for his promotion of the scientific conclusion that the earth rotates around the sun. This was deemed heretical by the Catholic Church. The church asserted that its view that the sun moved around the earth was an "absolute fact" based on scripture.[1] Science might say that the earth was not the center of the universe, but the church would reject or deny that fact.

Why did the Catholic Church prosecute Galileo? The church did so because church doctrine held that everything revolved around the earth. Galileo's scientific work challenged that doctrine and, by extension, the power of the church. Scientific observations are potentially very powerful, and power is inherently political. Where a scientific observation may contradict the "reality" most beneficial to those who compete in the political arena, resistance to science, science denial, and anti-science propaganda are typically weaponized to defend a political interest that may be threatened by facts.

Where scientific discovery arrives at conclusions that run contrary to cultural beliefs and values, human societies will easily resist or deny the science in favor of belief. Once upon a time, ancient Babylonian priests taught that lunar eclipses were caused by the restlessness of the gods. They were seen as signs that the gods were displeased with their kings. Local astronomers were eventually able to demonstrate that eclipses had a natural cause. This scientific discovery did not change the superstitious beliefs of the priests or all of the people. The human capacity to employ reason is a gift, one might say. But all too often, human beings use their "gift" of reason to justify a belief or a prejudice. This is a phenomenon known as *motivated reasoning*. Motivated reasoning, in both the political and cultural contexts, often makes it very difficult for facts to prevail.

Politics and culture inevitably influence how the observations and discoveries of science may be perceived in any society. Cultural or religious values and beliefs, subjective political values, and public perceptions of authority are part of the environment in which scientific information is received. This often contributes to the battle lines that are formed by the inevitable gap separating how science understands the world from how politics and people act in the world. This gap, observable throughout human history, may be especially troublesome in a time of a global public health crisis. In other words, a pandemic is a time when science must prevail over politics and self-interest. Culture and politics may work against that. Before we can begin to assess the American response to COVID-19, we must consider the cultural and political contexts in which that response took place.

In the United States today, there is a basic political reality that may be seen to impede the process of cooperation required to prepare for and respond to a pandemic. In the present-day context of American political life, all facts have become a matter of partisan dispute. A pandemic should not be a partisan issue. Everyone might well agree with that. But in the United States today, everything is partisan, and everything is weaponized for partisan warfare. The average citizen is bombarded daily with contentious misinformation from various special interests, politicians, partisan news coverage on cable television, and ideological trolls on social media. There is a declining public respect for public officials, public institutions, private institutions, and a near total mistrust of the media. While respect for science may be said to remain fairly high, there is nevertheless a considerable disagreement on the degree to which "expertise" should be trusted or valued in our public affairs. But then, Americans have never been overwhelmingly impressed by experts.

The American Cultural Context in 2020

Alexis de Tocqueville, known to all students of U.S. history as the author of *Democracy in America*, spent nine months traveling the United States in 1831. Tocqueville and Gustave de Beaumont had been sent to the United States by the French government to study the American prison system. But Tocqueville had another purpose in mind. He wanted to collect information about American society, including its religious, political, and economic character. In other words, Tocqueville and Beaumont used their official business as a pretext to study American society instead. Both men, it seems, had an intense interest in studying the new American experiment in democracy. Tocqueville had an intense interest in how religion and the notion of political liberty were combined in the United States in a manner that was uncommon in Europe. Tocqueville found much to admire about democracy in the United States, and he saw the ills of that democracy that needed to be addressed. Indeed, it was the excesses that he saw as inherent in democracy that suggested the likely potential for its self-destruction.

American democracy, as we were all instructed in our school days, is based on the foundation of popular sovereignty. "We the people" are the legitimate source of the legislative power that is exercised by our elected representatives. While citizens may be the source of sovereignty, Tocqueville's observations told him that they were generally disinterested in and separated from the social and political realms. He observed that Americans were mostly inclined to withdraw from society as a whole and retreat into a circle of family and friends. Tocqueville's observations in the United States suggested to him that there were three main threats to the American system of democracy: tyranny of the majority, individualism, and despotism.[2] Of particular interest in relation to an understanding of American culture is individualism. Tocqueville saw what he described as individualism to be unique to the United States. He observed that of all people he had studied, Americans seemed unique in that they felt no debt to the past and had no sense of obligation for the future. In assessing the world and arriving at their own conclusions about it, Americans felt no need to appeal to any authority outside of their own individual mind. To Tocqueville, Americans seemed to be lacking in what he called "public spirit."[3] Lacking public spirit, or having lost the inclination to band together to be involved in public affairs, Tocqueville warned that Americans may become too dependent on the state to do for them what they, joining and collaborating with their fellows, could do for themselves. Such disengagement would no doubt mean too little attention paid by citizens to their government, and this could only weaken the sovereign public's ability to hold its elected representatives accountable. It was also a danger that an uninformed and disengaged majority might come to support, explicitly or tacitly, measures that would harm the individual liberties of others.

Tocqueville's observations seem to be relevant as one examines American life today. Ours is indeed a very individualistic culture. Our politics is a battle between conflicting interests to advance their self-interests in public policy. In this battle, many Americans do not readily see how achieving a good for someone else may be connected to their own good. It is a competition. In this competition, we all too quickly lose the capacity to see differing interests as being interrelated.[4]

American individualism is the defining characteristic of the nation. It pretty much defines how most American lives are lived. Most average citizens are wrapped up in microsocial relations with family and like-minded friends. They do not interact much with "others." They avoid or ignore macrosocial relations with big government and big business. People may feel in control of their microsocial lives but be totally unaware of how their lives are being manipulated or impacted by the macrosocial world. Americans tend not to participate much in the larger world. Occasionally, they may vote or watch the news, but just as often, they see such things as being unimportant to them.[5]

In addition to individualism, there is another major cultural variable that more or less defines the American experience. Anti-intellectualism is indisputably a part of America's cultural heritage. In fact, anti-intellectualism is celebrated in some prominent political quarters. The celebration of anti-intellectualism, to the degree that it allows people to be ignorant without being stigmatized, aids in the creation of an atmosphere in which people can be influenced to embrace ideas that have absolutely no grounding in facts. This makes it much easier to create alternate and conflicting universes and increases the probability that Americans will live in different and incompatible worlds.

In his Pulitzer Prize–winning book, *Anti-Intellectualism in American Life*, Richard Hofstadter saw anti-intellectualism as something that was baked into American culture. He defined *anti-intellectualism* as a "resentment of the life of the mind. It is also a resentment of those who are considered to represent it."[6] He noted that there was, and always has been, an American disposition to constantly minimize the value of that life. This disposition was married to what Hofstadter saw as American utilitarianism. According to the utilitarian paradigm, a person's interactions with the world are guided by the principle of utility maximization. Rational thought and rational behavior are defined by the individual human actor as thoughts and actions that contribute to the enhancement of human utility (defined as pleasures) and the minimization of pain. The maximization of individual well-being, or self-interest, is the thing valued most by the utilitarian mind. Knowledge is not good in itself. It is good only insofar as it contributes to the enhancement of the welfare, subjectively defined, of individuals.

The preferred way of exercising the mind, according to Hofstadter, is mechanical. The utilitarian mind sees knowledge as being related to the performance of tasks and the making of decisions that contribute something of value to the human individual. This is usually thought of in materialistic terms. For example, Americans learn at an early age that they are defined by their station in life or the jobs they hold. They are taught that the value of their existence is defined in terms of the monetary rewards and material benefits they accumulate. For too many, this leads to the unfortunate conclusion that knowledge, such as it may seem useful to them, is practical and of use only in relation to the goal of individual material self-advancement. This is defined as *practicality* and is to be highly valued as the purpose of learning.[7]

It must be noted that anti-intellectualism does not mean a lack of intelligence. It must also be noted that even very intelligent people often embrace or exalt in ignorance. At the same time, it must be observed that the combination of anti-intellectualism and utilitarianism in American culture plants some seeds that may be destructive to the role that knowledge might ideally play in the guiding of our actions. Anti-intellectualism and utilitarianism often combine to justify placing the immediate and material interests of self ahead of everything else. They may combine to ignore the evidence at hand that contradicts our wants or beliefs. They may combine to elevate the importance of opinion in all things and to de-emphasize any of the objective facts we find to be inconvenient. When they together combine with our respect for the precious right of individuals to think for themselves, they may lead to the conclusion that one's opinion is as valid as another's knowledge in deciding the things that matter.

From the time Hofstadter published his prize-winning book in 1963 to the present, it can be said that American culture has been characterized by the accelerating and almost complete dismissal of science, the arts, and humanities as the measure for knowledge. These things are no longer, if they ever really were, the foundation for opinion. They have been replaced by other things (e.g., faith, ideology, conspiracy theories, entertainment, self-righteousness, ignorance, gullibility) as the justification for the opinions we hold. The digital age guaranteed that the dismissal of knowledge as the foundation for opinion would become almost complete. According to Max Bauerlein, author of *The Dumbest Generation*, the result has been a collective loss of history and context.[8]

The digital age has brought us the potential to increase opportunities for education, cultural activity, and political activism. It has also rapidly enhanced the opportunities to make us dumber. In an age when we have more information at our fingertips than any previous generation, we also have an unprecedented lack of respect for knowledge-based or expert analysis that is available online. We are in fact less and less able to identify legitimate and expert sources of information and too easily drawn to a wealth of misinformation. There is a limitless supply of junk on the internet and our social media. It actually overwhelms legitimate information and expert analysis. While this may or may not make us dummies, it most certainly creates a world in which reasoned, informed, and intelligent thought is more difficult to convey.

In our republic, political leaders must try to form a governing coalition among people and interests who hold competing views and are pursuing different self-interests. This is very difficult to do, even when everyone agrees on the underlying facts that define reality. When reasoned, informed, and intelligent thought and dialogue are not possible, agreement on what is real (the underlying facts) is not possible. This is a potentially fatal flaw in any political system that relies on an informed and sovereign citizenry to hold it accountable. When public misperceptions outweigh knowledge as the driving force in our public discourse, science will be hard put to compete.

Valuing the work of intellectuals, including scientists, is absolutely essential for a well-functioning republic such as the United States. An informed and well-educated citizenry is an indispensable necessity in any successful democracy. When something as serious and threatening as a global pandemic occurs, the ability of the citizenry and their leaders to apply the expert knowledge of the scientific community to the task of responding to the crisis and mitigating its harms is an essential necessity, or so one would think. Politics will still happen, and disputes over matters of importance will not go away.

Ideally, in a pandemic scenario, the objective scientific experts would be seen as the rational and authoritative arbiters of public disputes over scientific or technical issues. But this is to assume something that cannot be taken for granted in the United States today. It assumes that something will matter more than politics and partisan conflict during a global public health emergency. But the evolution of tribalism, or extreme partisan division, in American politics has shaped and defined public perceptions of all things. Everything, including a pandemic, is political in the United States.

During the first wave of the COVID-19 outbreak in the United States, public opinion surveys showed that Americans did have an increased trust for scientific and medical experts. But when broken down along partisan lines, there were notable differences (see table 3.1). Differences of opinion about science and scientific expertise are not new developments in American public opinion. In 2016, according to a Pew Research Center survey, only 24 percent of Americans indicated that they had a great deal of confidence that medical scientists acted in the best interests of the American people. In 2020, as the COVID-19 crisis became real, that confidence level increased to 53 percent. But, as table 3.1 shows, that increase was primarily among Democrats and not Republicans.

Table 3.1   Percent of U.S. Adults Who Have a Great Deal of Confidence in Medical Scientists to Act in the Best Interests of the Public

	All Adults	Republicans	Democrats
2016	24%	____	____
2019	35%	32%	37%
2020	43%	31%	53%

Source: Pew Research Center, June 3, 2020, https://www.pewresearch.org/science /2020/06/03/partisan-differences-over-the-pandemic-response-are-growing/ps_2020 -06-03_sci-am-trust_00-1/

One might look at federal spending on research and development as a window into the American commitment to science. It is often said that a nation's spending on R & D as a share of the gross domestic product is an excellent gauge of a nation's capacity for innovation. Such spending has been trending downward in the United States in recent years. Surveys have identified a partisan gap in the United States when it comes to support for more governmental funding for scientific research.[9] In 2001, there was no significant divide between Democrats and Republicans with respect to support of government spending for scientific research. In subsequent years, Republican support trended steadily downward before going up a bit more recently. Democratic support has remained relatively steady for more than a decade, and in the past couple of years, it has risen significantly.[10]

Observations such as these are no surprise. Over the past two decades, partisan polarization has been the most powerful force driving public opinion. On virtually every issue one can think of, partisan differences are wider today than at any time in the memory of any living American. The divide between Republicans and Democrats on fundamental values related to the role of government, the environment, race, immigration, and all other issues has become so complete that there is little common ground left and almost no room for compromise.

Partisan differences are an inevitable part of political life in a free society, and they are often a constructive thing if they contribute to a spirited and informed exchange of views that stimulates citizens to participate and promote the principled views that they hold. But when partisanship is not accompanied by the civilizing effect of knowledge or the restraint of objective fact, where it is literally all there is, it can be very difficult for expertise to be heard and valued for what it is. Like everything else, it will be politicized, and the public will make of it whatever their ideological or partisan preferences want it to be.

Table 3.2   Partisan Differences on the Role of Testing and Spread of Coronavirus

Social distancing measures are helping a lot to slow the spread of coronavirus

Republicans 47%   Democrats 76%   All U.S. adults 59%

Coronavirus spreads more easily than other infectious viruses

Republicans 58%   Democrats 78%   All U.S. adults 68%

There is not enough testing for coronavirus

Republicans 31%   Democrats 82%   All U.S. adults 58%

Not enough people are following social distancing measures

Republicans 36%   Democrats 72%   All U.S. adults 57%

Source: Pew Research Center, June 2, 2020, https://www.pewresearch.org/science/2020/06/03/partisan-differences-over-the-pandemic-response-are-growing/ps_2020-06-03_sci-am-trust_00-3/

As COVID-19 spread across the nation, Americans were exposed to the best expert scientific analysis. They were informed about the disease and how easily the virus would spread. They were informed about the importance of defensive measures like social distancing. They were all exposed to the same information from valid sources. They were also exposed to other things that we shall examine in the next chapter. But as table 3.2 shows, once again, Americans reacted along partisan lines.

Why do these partisan differences about scientific matters exist? Why is one partisan group more likely to be supportive of and trusting of science than the other? The answers to these questions require some assessment of the political landscape in the United States. Just as our cultural values borne of our tradition of anti-intellectualism and utilitarian logic influence our opinions, so too do the partisan values and the political wars we have about them shape our thinking. Both, as we shall see, make it more and more difficult to arrive at objective conclusions about the events and fundamental realities that life brings to our doorstep. Both may be seen to influence our thinking even during something as objectively real as a global pandemic.

The Political Context of 2020

Republicans and Democrats in the United States are further apart ideologically than at any point in recent history. Recent surveys show that a growing number of Republicans and Democrats hold highly negative views of each other. They see each other as enemies. The partisan antipathy that has risen in recent decades has made compromises across party lines, once viewed as the basic necessity for governing, increasingly difficult.[11] Some would say it has made compromise impossible. "Ideological silos," socializing only with people who share one's views, have become more common. To partisans on both sides, right and left, compromise now means always getting everything they want. Failing that, the next best result is to inconvenience or frustrate the other side.[12]

Democrats and Republicans agree on less and less, but that is not the biggest concern. On a more basic level, they do not accept the same facts as the starting point for debate. They do not share a reality. Too frequently, they occupy an antirational world in which every fact is suspect, every rational thought is the enemy's trick, and critical thinking is unholy or unpatriotic. Reality itself is reduced to a matter of partisan perception uninfluenced by any objective foundation in fact or truth. Politically, the United States has become sorted into two teams. The driving force in American politics is the contempt these two teams have for each other. Americans are less and less able to understand, communicate, or empathize with the other side. Hyperpolarization has become the new political norm.

Anger and divisiveness are nothing new in American politics, but they have become so intense in recent years that they have produced an unhealthy anxiety in the culture. Differences of opinion concerning the most provocative issues (e.g., illegal immigration, race, health care, procreation, foreign relations) have seen the political left and the political right coalescing around dramatically opposing and irreconcilable worldviews. Stubborn intractability in contemporary American politics has left many feeling more vulnerable and confused. It has caused some of those feeling most vulnerable and afraid to embrace what can only be described as authoritarian preferences.[13] The net result seems to be the paralysis of government and the abandonment of public policy as an effective tool to serve the broader public interest.

With respect to science generally, partisan divisions became more acute beginning in the decade of the 1960s. As Shawn Otto explains it in his monumental book *The War on Science*, the advances in human control of the reproductive cycle and the birth of environmental science began to reshape the playing field. With the advance of the birth control pill and the legalization of abortion in 1973 (*Roe v. Wade*), religious conservatives saw advances in the biological sciences as offensive to their faith and to the will of God. With advances in environmental science and the explosion of a new environmental movement that it inspired, energy, chemical, and agricultural industries were equally offended by what they saw as an infringement on their unrestricted right to make money.[14] This resulted in a new political alliance that reshaped conservative politics. Religious conservatives and fundamentalists found themselves in bed with major industries. The religious right's opposition to contraception, abortion, in vitro fertilization, and governmental policies to promote procreation rights combined with the corporate industrial opposition to government regulations and the felt need to protect corporate freedom to form a marriage of convenience. On a host of issues (e.g., climate change, smoking, evolution, sex education, gun control, acid rain), industrial and religious vested interests were willing to forge an anti-government alliance of convenience and collaborate, or use each other, to resist the power of government. Both were also ready to resist or deny any science that worked against their respective interests.[15] Freedom, corporate or religious, was being threatened by government in the eyes of the partners in this marriage. Defense of freedom was the self-defined purpose of this union on the political right. Government was the enemy.

Another marriage of convenience formed on the political left. The groups that constituted the environmental movement, pro-choice women, and progressives were generally drawn to the environmental scientists and medical researchers in appreciation of their ongoing work. Whether it was freedom of choice or freedom from dangerous chemical exposure, the basis of this progressive marriage with science was freedom. While generally more supportive of scientific research than the political right, the left also has its moments when its ideological preferences bring it into opposition with science. Suspicions of hidden dangers to their health and well-being, usually perceived to be of corporate design, have caused many progressives to support notions not supported by scientific evidence (e.g., cell phones cause brain cancer, vaccines cause autism, genetically modified crops are unsafe to eat).[16] While more common on the political right, both left and right will deny science when it suits their partisan desires.

Science denial on the political right begins with the assumption that liberal scientists have a socialist agenda and that they are seeking more money from the government so that they can control or regulate your life and limit your freedom. Science denial from the political left is aimed at impersonal doctors, greedy drug manufacturers and corporations, and mechanistic scientists who seek to hide dangers to our safety and health to maximize their profits. None of the assumptions, from the right or the left, have anything to do with science, of course. In fact, scientists do not really inform either. Scientific research is not always a variable that ideological combatants rigorously consult in arriving at their conclusions.

The denial of science has been a constant theme in political discourse for almost all of our history. It has been muted a bit at times, when science has been deemed essential to deal with a crisis, but it has always been there. The chemical industry, always with an eye on its bottom line, attacked Rachel Carson after she published *Silent Spring* in 1962. Anti-science attacks against environmental science from business interests (e.g., cigarette manufacturers, the oil and gas industry) escalated throughout the 1960s and beyond. Corporations worried about profits began to see scientific research as a threat to their interests. Conservative evangelicals ramped up attacks on evolution in the 1990s and 2000s, and we see state legislatures promoting their agenda even today. The anti-vax movement began around the same time.[17]

We must be careful to note that the majority of Americans are not science deniers or anti-science. But those who are can be extremely vocal, especially on social media. One ironic result is that science and technology have increased their effectiveness in attacking the science they wish to deny. Politicians get into the science denial act as well. Corporate dollars that support science denial also support and use politicians to pursue their interests. Politicians want the corporate dollars to fund their campaigns. All of this translates into making our public dialogue, and our political discourse, a contest between the demand for more evidence-based decision-making and a retreat into non-evidence-based, corporately designed, and religious or quasi-religious alternatives.

Political actors, at all levels of government, view scientific research as something that can be useful when it supports the specific goals or causes they wish to advance. At the same time, where scientific research may be at odds with the preferences of policy makers and the vested interests that support them, it is very quickly deep-sixed or delegitimized in the fact-free zone of partisan political discourse.[18] Even when they basically agree on a scientific matter, partisanship often gets in the way of addressing it in a constructive way.

During the Obama administration, a bipartisan group of members of Congress sponsored a bill that would have created a U.S. science laureate. The position would have been honorary and unpaid. As such, there would be no fuss over budgets or funding. The purpose was to appoint a science laureate who would be tasked with encouraging U.S. schoolchildren to pursue careers in science. The passage of this proposal, which had support from the leadership of both parties, seemed to be a sure thing. But the bill would be dropped from the docket when the American Conservative Union (ACU), a right-wing activist group, expressed concerns that President Obama could not be trusted to make such an appointment. The group warned that he might appoint a "liberal" scientist who might sway public opinion on issues such as climate change.[19] Even when they agree, policy makers are likely to disagree where science is concerned.

Many observers have noted that politicians, especially on the political right, do not reject or deny science for what it says. They reject or deny it for what it implies. *Implicatory denial* means that people reject scientific evidence not because there is anything wrong with the science but because they do not like its implications with respect to policy options or actions that the evidence suggests but their ideology abhors. So much of what sound scientific research discovers is unwelcome in partisan quarters. Why? Because scientific evidence in areas such as environmental science and public health often points to the need for government interventions to address the problem. Conservatives in particular react negatively to that because it often conflicts with their anti-regulatory ideology and their preference for limited government. This dynamic has been particularly potent in the efforts to cast doubt about the work of climate scientists. Naomi Oreskes and Erik Conway portray this dynamic in exquisite detail in their 2010 book, *Merchants of Doubt*.[20]

Corporate interests spend unlimited amounts of money and political propagandists spew unlimited amounts of verbiage to discredit legitimate science. They see this as being essential in the pursuit of their material or ideological interests. Their primary objective is to create such doubt about the work scientific researchers do that it detracts from the legitimacy of their findings.[21] This not only spreads misinformation about scientific matters but also causes serious conflict within the body politic. The efforts to discredit the scientific consensus about climate change, for example, have sharpened the partisan divide and made science itself a target for some partisans. Climate scientists have faced threats of violence for the work they do. Michael E. Mann, a renowned climate scientist at Penn State University, publicly shared his experiences in 2016. He noted that he had "faced hostile investigations by politicians, demands for me to be fired from my job, threats against my life and even threats against my family."[22] Many people today seem to believe that scientists are biased in their work and that they are pursing ideological rather than scientific objectives. It was not always thus, but this public perception has been exquisitely manufactured by the corporate and fundamentalist science deniers who have joined forces to discredit science as a means of advancing their causes and interests.

Until about the mid-twentieth century, scientific knowledge was considered by most Americans to be dependable and unbiased. In fact, it was regarded as a source of objective truth by policy makers and citizens alike.[23] The logic of this perception seemed self-evident to all. Scientific experts, whose academic and professional credentials were the unquestionable foundation of their legitimacy and integrity, advised the policy makers, and the policy makers rarely questioned the legitimacy of the advice they received. A person who grew up in the 1960s, the age of the space race and the moon landing, was routinely impressed by the value of science and believed in its wonderous capacity to improve the world. But since that time, this dynamic has changed dramatically. The issues and controversies entering the political arena—combined with the intensification of ideological and partisan differences over the decades since that time—have created greater distance between politics and science. These developments have increased the tension and created unhealthy conflicts between the conclusions reached by scientific experts and the values of ideological policy makers, citizens, and laypeople.[24]

Consider, for a moment, some of the things we have seen (if we were actually paying attention) over the past decade alone that tell us that science is just another political football to be kicked around. We have witnessed the many highly partisan debates about things such as stem cell research, vaccines, evolution, and anthropogenic climate change. We have heard many competing and irreconcilable claims made by scientists, special interests, and members of Congress. Strategically manipulated questions have been aimed with partisan precision to cast doubt on the reliability of scientific research and testimony. We saw a U.S. senator stand up in the well of the Senate and smugly hold up a snowball as his proof that climate change is a hoax. We have seen corporations and special interests funding pseudoscience reports that support their vested interests by muddying the waters around legitimate science. We have seen the misinterpretation and exaggeration of the meaning of legitimate scientific disagreement and unresolved questions for the sole purpose of skewing it to provide more cover for those who only wish to deny what science actually does know. The culmination of this symphony of distortion may be best summed up with the words of one member of Congress as he responded to the testimony of a scientific expert with whom he disagreed. He uttered the immortal words that best describe the depth to which respect for science has sunk: "You have your science; I have mine."[25]

The inability of science to be understood for what it objectively is and the interpretation of its results through the lens of partisanship reduces its ability to influence our public decision makers or to inform public behavior. Take climate change denial as an example. Climate change denial persists in the face of accumulating evidence and a strengthening scientific consensus. In some segments of the American population, we have seen, as one might expect, increased acceptance of the science regarding climate change. But there is a significant segment of the population for which the exact opposite is true. Among many hard-core conservatives and free market advocates, one finds that as the scientific consensus has been solidified by irrefutable evidence, climate change denial has remained steady or even increased. This response is driven, according to various empirical studies, by the expectation that climate scientists have been falsifying data to support the assertions being made about the dangers or threats posed by climate change.[26] This is a thought pattern that psychologists tell us is associated with conspiratorial thinking. Conspiratorial thinking is immune to new evidence. In fact, any new evidence that disproves the conspiracy is immediately viewed as a part of the conspiracy.[27] When a significant portion of the public believes that scientific research is part of a conspiracy, it is hard to see how science can avoid being dragged into the political cross fire.

The number of people ideologically predisposed to reject science in favor of politics is large enough to have altered the nature of public discourse and to influence the outcomes of elections. This is especially true among Republicans. A Republican candidate is likely to be propelled by a strong anti-science wind. This appeals to the conservative base, and it also results in the election of officeholders who themselves are full-fledged science deniers. Anti-science rhetoric has become normalized in present-day American politics, and it has become a staple among conservative officeholders. Examples abound. Congressman Paul Broun (R-GA) told a luncheon audience, "All that stuff I was taught about evolution and embryology, big bang theory, all that is lies straight from the pit of hell."[28] Congressman John Shimkus (R-IL), chairman of the House Subcommittee on Environment and the Economy and a climate change denier, cited the Bible as his source for rejecting science. He said, while waving his Bible in a congressional hearing, "The earth will end only when God says its time is over." He went on to proclaim, based on theological argument, that "this is a carbon-starved planet."[29] The person elected to the U.S. presidency in 2016, Donald Trump, tweeted in 2014, "Snowing in Texas and Louisiana, record setting freezing temperatures throughout the country and beyond. Global warming is an expensive hoax!"[30] Clearly, being anti-science is not a handicap in electoral politics in the United States.

It would seem obvious that in the middle of a serious global pandemic that science denial, or anti-science bias, is the last thing one would hope to see driving human behavior. It is certainly not the thing that one would want to see driving governmental decision-making. Yet, at the height of the COVID-19 outbreak in the United States, the nation's leading infectious disease expert, Dr. Anthony Fauci, suggested that a pervasive "anti-science bias" led many Americans to disregard the advice of public health experts. He expressed concerns about people willingly ignoring science despite obvious risks to their health. He cited an anti-science bias among people that predisposed them not to believe authorities during the crisis. This he called "inconceivable." He added, "That's unfortunate because, you know, science is truth."[31] Frankly, and not to detract from the point Dr. Fauci tried to make in his remarks, the anti-science bias he observed was not inconceivable. Given the anti-intellectualism in American culture and the existing political climate in the United States in the years leading up to the pandemic, it was absolutely predictable and should have been anticipated.

Science and technology may sometimes lead us astray (often due to some commercial interests manipulating things). One famous example involves early studies that linked fat consumption to heart disease. The massive influx of trans fats and carbohydrates to the American diet had the exact opposite effect. It resulted in much worse health, and the lobbying by trans fat producers was part of the reason this happened. People frequently cite situations such as these when questioning science.

For the most part, science and technology are concerned with reality. It may be observed that there are always going to be aspects of reality that are unpopular. In the United States, some people deny climate change science because it is difficult to shoulder the financial burden. Some people do not believe in evolution because it contradicts their religious beliefs. Some people do not support fluoridation because chemicals are scary. In other words, science sometimes causes people to choose between emotions and scientific consensus on what is actually happening, and too many people choose emotions. Some people dislike science because they feel like scientists, and those with postgraduate degrees, look down on and belittle those with less education. Some are offended by this and react by finding a class of people (an educated scientific elite) and their expertise to be a threat. Some people just do not like what science may be telling them. They simply do not want to believe and will not accept the changes that science tells them are coming because it means their ideas of how life should be lived on earth might be wrong. It also threatens them with the thought that their ideas about their future might be wrong as well. Change is pretty scary, and some people want to blame the providers of the news about changes they do not like to hear about for their unease or fear. All of this is normal in the American cultural experience. When you add to this the partisan toxicity of American politics over the past few decades, one has a perfect anti-science storm gathering.

In advance of the 2020 election in the United States, public opinion surveys found major partisan divisions of the electorate where matters of science were concerned. More Democrats than Republicans believed that the scientific method produced accurate conclusions. Republicans were more likely than Democrats to view scientists as susceptible to bias. Democrats were also more likely to think that scientific experts were better at making decisions about scientific issues than other people. Democrats more so than Republicans valued the opinions of scientific experts on policy matters.[32] It should be no surprise to find that some partisan differences over the science and its role in the pandemic response would show growing divisions between Republicans and Democrats in the confidence they have in medical scientists. All these findings suggest that the role of leadership, especially at the national level, would be critical to articulate and successfully implement a coherent national strategy to respond to a global pandemic. Gaining public confidence and cooperation in that effort would not be easy.

Conclusion: The Leadership Challenge

As the forty-fifth president of the United States took office in January 2017, partisan divisions in the nation were arguably at a fever pitch. More important, the new president was not exactly committed, in contrast to his two immediate predecessors, to the notion that a national commitment to science is essential for our prosperity, our security, our health, our environment, and our quality of life. Indeed, he demonstrated with swiftness and precision that science would be treated as an obstacle to be overcome by his administration. The very moment he took the oath of office, all mention of climate change was removed from the White House web page. One agency in particular was singled out. On day three of the new presidency, the Environmental Protection Agency (EPA) was barred from posting updates on social media or providing any information to the press. Just a few days later, the administration mandated that all EPA studies first be reviewed by political staffers at the White House before being released to the public. This reversed an Obama administration rule that had allowed EPA scientists to work uncompromised by political interference. And this was just the beginning.

In March 2017, the new Trump administration proposed cutting the EPA budget by 25 percent. This proposal would not be approved, but the signal was clear. The new administration was determined to scale back, if not eliminate, the EPA's role in protecting the environment. Soon the new administration would withdraw an Obama-era request that oil and natural gas companies provide information on their methane emissions. The newly appointed and confirmed EPA administrator, Scott Pruitt, made headlines when he said he did not believe that carbon dioxide was a "primary contributor to global warming."[33] By April 2017, the administration was scuttling the efforts of the EPA to reduce the emission of toxic chemicals. At this same time, the administration fired the eighteen-member Board of Scientific Counselors, a panel of evaluators who reviewed all the work done by EPA scientists. This panel had been specifically created to assist government regulators in developing the most scientifically sound rules to protect clean air, water, and soil, among many other things.[34]

On June 1, 2017, Donald Trump's resistance to climate science (he had called climate change a "hoax" during the 2016 campaign) culminated in his decision to withdraw the United States from the historic 2015 Paris climate accord. The speed and intensity with which the new administration was seeking to limit, control, and outright deny science was considered to be unprecedented.[35] This caused a strong reaction within the scientific community. Unofficial Twitter accounts were launched to voice resistance to the Trump administration's quick succession of orders and decisions aimed at limiting the influence of science. Some were tweeting on behalf of unidentified federal scientists. Resistance among the professional scientists was rumored at the Park Service, NASA, the U.S. Forest Service, the EPA, and in several cabinet departments. In April 2017, a March for Science brought scientists and citizens to the streets of the nation's capital to respond to what was perceived as unprecedented attacks on science by the new administration.[36]

It should be noted that the new administration's disregard for and attacks on science, whether prompted by the political right's aversion to government regulation, by corporate and business special interests who fear their bottom line is negatively impacted by objective scientific research, by fundamentalist religious groups, or by various conspiracy theories that suggest scientists are a part of some left-wing plot to destroy capitalism and take away individual liberty, was a continuation of an unfortunate anti-science trend on the political right in the United States. But the new administration did represent a dramatic acceleration of that trend.

Just as this acceleration blasted into action in 2017, a new avian influenza strain reignited global concerns about a new pandemic. This was the H7N9 virus that was spreading across China and mainly infecting poultry. But it had spread from chickens to humans, and nine in ten humans who became infected with it came down with pneumonia. Seventy-five percent of the infected humans experienced severe respiratory problems and ended up in intensive care. Over 40 percent of infected humans died.[37] H7N9 was China's fifth-largest outbreak of avian influenza. The world was watching closely, and the experts once again expressed the importance of monitoring and being prepared.

So, 2017 began with news of a heightened risk of a global pandemic. The new Trump administration had not yet appointed, and would not soon, senior officials to head the key federal agencies responsible for pandemic preparedness. This meant there were leadership vacancies in the Department of Health and Human Services (HHS), the National Institutes for Health (NIH), and the Centers for Disease Control and Prevention (CDC). In addition to the vacancies, the new administration was proposing deep budget cuts for these agencies (including a $5.8 billion reduction in NIH biomedical research funding). Not all of these cuts were approved, but the administration's objectives were abundantly clear.[38] The NIH plays an essential role in detecting outbreaks of new viruses, supporting research to develop vaccines, conducting international health research, and containing the spread of any outbreak that might occur.[39] Any reasonably informed individual aware of the growing global concerns about pandemic preparedness, the experiences of the two previous administrations in dealing with this concern, and how "political" science had become in an increasingly toxic political environment would have to be very concerned about recent events. Leadership vacancies and proposed budget cuts in the agencies that are responsible for the nation's health security would not be reassuring to one who understood that the pandemic risk meter was on high alert around the globe. Of even greater concern to many of those who might be aware of all of this, one might suppose, was the apparent lack of commitment by the new administration to science at a time when it could be most important. In a pandemic, it could be the difference between life and death for many.

The inexorable logic of any contagious virus is that it spreads. Urban density, mass transit, and large assemblies of people are among the things that will provide a vector in some places. But a virus will not be particular when all is said and done. Any human interaction in any place or context will do. The virus will spread. A pandemic describes an infectious disease where we see a significant and ongoing person-to-person spread in multiple countries around the world at the same time. Pandemics are more likely if a virus is brand new, able to easily infect people, and can spread from person to person in an efficient and sustained way. In 2020, the new coronavirus would tick all these boxes.

With no vaccine or treatment to prevent or cure COVID-19 as it swept across the globe, containing its spread would be the most vital thing that needed to be done. This would require that science and our political leadership were prepared and efficient, informed, and ready to act together in a timely, orderly, and unified response. The fight against a pandemic virus cannot be waged in an environment infected with misinformation and a cloud of confusion. It cannot be waged if partisan political preferences remain so intense that they contribute to the rejection of scientific evidence or doubts about the severity of the crisis. And it cannot be waged if political leadership remains political. In a pandemic, leadership is about science and morality, not party or ideology. It is perhaps a revealing insight into the state of the world that as the COVID-19 pandemic was in full swing, the World Health Organization (WHO) found it necessary to warn nations about the danger of "politicizing" the pandemic. The WHO felt compelled to remind us that political divisions would harm any chances for a proper and effective pandemic response.[40]

In a politically divided United States in 2020, the task of leadership would be more critical than ever. In a culture as individualistic and suspicious of both scientific expertise and political leadership as the United States can be at times, leadership would be difficult. Even with the proper reliance on science and the availability of expertise to guide them, political leaders will find themselves tested to the limit of their abilities. A pandemic crisis is a time when their competence, integrity, and personality must rise to new levels. The good news was that as the new administration began its work in 2017, a battle plan for leadership during a pandemic had been developed. It needed refinement, perhaps, but there was a good place to begin. The bad news was that the new administration seemed disinterested in beginning. It would not be unreasonable to wonder whether our national leadership was adequately prepared to lead during a global pandemic. That would be a reasonable thing to wonder about with respect to any administration of either party. With respect to the Trump administration, 2020 would be the end of the wondering. The question of how well prepared we were and the question of leadership would both be answered with certainty and absolute clarity.

CHAPTER FOUR

The End of Wondering: The First Wave Hits the United States

"I wish it need not have happened in my time," said Frodo. "So do I," said Gandalf, "and so do all who live in such times. But that is not for them to decide. All we have to decide is what to do with the time that is given us."
—J. R. R. Tolkien

"Where are we going Pooh?" "Home Piglet. We're going home because that's the best thing to do right now."
—A. A. Milne

Introduction

The day after his inauguration as the forty-fifth president of the United States, Donald Trump was obsessed, as always, with himself. He had not felt that the media and the movers and shakers in the nation's capital had welcomed his coronation with the appropriate enthusiasm. He was somewhat disappointed with the absence of star power at the concert that had taken place at the Lincoln Memorial. He was angry that the nation's intelligence community had concluded that the Russians had interfered in the 2016 election to his advantage, and he was increasingly irate at stories emerging about his own nefarious relationships with Russians. In short, he did not enjoy his inauguration. His inaugural speech, a combative and truculent presentation describing an American carnage unseen by anyone else, struck a strange note to say the least. Not only was it not considered great oratory by most observers, but it was also summed up most eloquently by former president George W. Bush as "some weird shit."[1] The next day, as he assumed the great burdens of his office, the new president made his priorities clear.

The first order of business in the Trump White House was to replace a series of inspirational photographs in the West Wing with images of crowd scenes at his inaugural ceremony. He had been chattering nonstop with aides and in phone calls with friends about the "big crowds." He saw over a million people who were not there and proclaimed the crowds to be the largest to have ever attended a presidential inaugural. He had his new press secretary, Sean Spicer, spend the entire day defending that assertion before the media. Of course, he spent a good deal of his own time tweeting about the historic size of his crowds.[2] All evidence to the contrary was said to be "fake news" produced by a hostile mainstream media. Whatever else each day brought to the president's attention, priority one was always to control the narrative of the day, place himself in the center of attention, and win the news cycle. Perhaps all presidents do that to some extent, but none had ever done it to the extent and with the intensity of this president. It was close to his sole focus. He did not feel that he had to worry about the details of governing because he was, as he saw it, a "stable genius" with no need for experts to tell him what to do.

The new president frequently reminded the public of just how smart he was. He claimed to be an expert on every issue. When it came to the courts, he was quick to say, "I know more about courts than any human being on earth." With respect to ISIS, he provided assurance: "I know more about ISIS than the generals do." Technology, you ask? "Nobody knows more about technology than me." There was literally no issue or topic that he did not know more about than everybody else.[3]

Of course, the people who worked up close and personal with the president in the White House could tell you differently. They repeatedly saw the president speak incoherently or fall flat on his face when trying to discuss any of these matters of substance. The nation soon learned that his own top officials derided him as an "idiot" and a "moron" behind closed doors. For all of the president's self-proclaimed genius, most felt his level of understanding was that of a sixth grader or, in many instances, less.[4] To the endearing traits of craving constant attention and self-aggrandization, one more variable must be introduced as a critical descriptor of the Trump leadership style. He lies.

Most politicians evade the truth once in a while. In fact, all of us do. It is estimated that even the most honest among us—and let us assume we are all basically honest most of the time—will fib or stretch the truth a couple of times each day. An analysis published in *Forbes* in April 2020 evaluated the over eighteen thousand lies President Trump supposedly told (according to various fact checkers) during his presidency. In 2020, he was averaging 23.8 lies per day. The distribution of lies was of more interest than the sheer number. It was not a flat distribution. Instead, there were some topics that seemed to attract more efforts at presidential deception. These included the economy, guns, education, and elections. The persistent bouts of presidential lying on Twitter were also noteworthy. Presidential tweets traveled fast and were widely distributed. This made them difficult for facts (and fact checkers) to catch up with. Rally speeches, press briefings, and interviews were also expertly used to spread misinformation. It seemed as if the truth no longer had any ability to compete with lies in the public domain. In our partisan and divided political landscape, it was as if we had arrived at a place where the lie never died and the truth rarely won.[5]

The FBI investigation, and later the investigation by special prosecutor Robert S. Mueller, into the Russian interference in the 2016 election would see the president seek to impede the process, deny the truth of the findings, and perhaps even perjure himself in his written responses to the special prosecutor's questions. Many who read the complete Mueller report, both volumes, cover to cover were astonished at the obvious connections reported between the Russians and persons in the Trump campaign. Mueller concluded that the evidence was not strong enough to bring charges of a criminal conspiracy, but there was absolutely no doubt that there had been some collusion between the campaign and the Russians. Volume two clearly identified as many as ten instances of presidential obstruction of justice.

But there would be no public outcry demanding that the campaign or the president be held accountable for anything. Despite criminal convictions of lesser campaign staffers and associates, the Mueller report was effectively defanged and made irrelevant in the political arena by the manipulation of Attorney General William Barr and the effective misrepresentation of truth by the president ("no collusion—no obstruction") and his supporters. The fact remains that the Mueller report did outline disturbing evidence that was ignored or swept away.[6]

Whatever one's perspective or opinion about any of the points made in the preceding paragraphs, one thing must be made crystal clear in relation to the COVID-19 outbreak: President Trump's leadership style may not have been a good fit for a public health crisis. Selflessness, scientific knowledge, truthfulness, and accurate communication are the important leadership traits that matter most during a pandemic. Honesty without ambiguity, reliable fact-based communication, empathy, listening to experts, and humility are essential because of the need to unite our diverse (and divided) nation to manage a crisis. Political leadership during a pandemic—during any crisis for that matter—must strive to unite us. It tries to do this by recalling us to our shared values when circumstances may have made us forget them. Such leadership asks for our compassion, sacrifice, and love of neighbor and country.

A crisis with life-and-death consequences is not a time for politics as usual. It is not a time for leaders to worry about themselves or their political fortunes as a genuine disaster hits those they are supposed to serve and lead. Crisis leadership requires very different traits and behaviors than those on display throughout the Trump presidency. No matter how well or how poorly a nation may be prepared for the crisis, the ability of leaders to rise to the occasion and display the desired traits—or their inability or failure to do so—will greatly influence the successes or failures that follow.

Time Wasted as COVID-19 Approaches

Just two months before a new coronavirus began its deadly advance across the world, the Trump administration ended a $200 million pandemic early-warning program. This program, begun by the U.S. Agency for International Development in 2009, was aimed at training scientists in China and other countries to detect pandemic threats. The initiative, called PREDICT, trained and supported staff in sixty laboratories around the world. The work going on in these laboratories had already identified 1,200 different viruses, including 160 new coronaviruses, that had the potential to erupt into pandemics.[7] The PREDICT project was launched in response to the H5N1 scare of 2005–2006 and was considered to be a vital necessity in a world where the potential for new pandemic outbreaks is significantly increasing. Prediction is necessary for preparation and without preparation, there could be no effective response to a pandemic.

The elimination of the PREDICT program was criticized by many observers as a part of an ongoing Trump administration effort that had resulted in the downgrading of global health security.[8] Combined with other proposed budget cuts in federal public health agencies and programs, it seemed to verify the observation of critics that the Trump administration had significantly reduced the nation's focus on public health concerns.

Both the Bush and the Obama administrations had emphasized pandemic preparedness between 2005 and 2017. This culminated in the creation of a pandemic planning unit within the National Security Council (NSC). The National Security Council Directorate for Global Health Security and Biodefense created the pandemic playbook that had been passed on to the Trump administration. As discussed in chapter 2, this playbook was based on the premise that the federal government needed to be prepared to lead when a national public health crisis emerged. The plan stressed that it was critically important that the federal response be prepared to present a "unified message" to manage the American public's questions and concerns during a crisis. It was also imperative to provide direction to enhance state and local, as well as citizen, cooperation in implementing a coordinated and successful response to a pandemic. Early coordination of risk communication through a single federal spokesperson was also said to be critical.

All indications were that the Trump administration never consulted the playbook and never took seriously the need to work to perfect our planning for a pandemic. In 2018, the National Security Council Directorate for Global Health Security and Biodefense was eliminated by the Trump administration.

According to John Bolton, Trump's national security adviser in 2018, the decision to eliminate the NSC planning body was taken to reduce duplication and to enhance coordination and efficiency. The responsibilities of the NSC directorate dealing with global health and biodefense were reassigned to another directorate dealing with weapons of mass destruction. Bolton maintained that the personnel working on global health continued their work in the combined directorate.[9]

Others saw the elimination of the NSC planning group dedicated to health security and the combining of it with another directorate as the weakening of a focus that needed to be sharpened. At a time when the risks of a global pandemic were absolutely increasing, and after the preceding two administrations had recognized the need to sharpen both our preparation and the readiness of the federal government, the new directorate was considered essential to lead with a strong and consistent unified approach. The shelving of the pandemic playbook and the elimination of the NSC planning body seemed to lessen the urgency of the task and to remove it further from the center of the White House's attention than was advisable.

The logic of creating the new directorate had been based on the identification of a threat that needed to be separated and isolated from other concerns. It needed to be elevated to the center of attention. The decision to eliminate the new directorate only served to remove it from view and bury it in the mix of other concerns. It also moved pandemic preparedness further from the president's focus. Even with his paint-by-numbers bureaucratic defense of the move to eliminate the NSC directorate dealing with global health at a time when global health was under increasing threats, John Bolton admitted that the Trump administration was not prepared for COVID-19.[10]

As COVID-19 ambled its way across the globe and toward the United States, precious time was wasted. As it turns out, the Trump administration's response to the pandemic was doomed from the start. Its simplistic strategy at the outset was to keep COVID-19 out of the United States. Since early January 2020, epidemiologists and public health officials and experts had warned the president and the nation that believing his containment strategy could work was a grave mistake.[11] But then it is doubtful that President Trump ever fully appreciated what he would be dealing with as the pandemic approached American shores. Indeed, despite the warnings of the Centers for Disease Control and Prevention (CDC) and other federal agencies that the threat was growing and that we needed to be prepared to respond quickly to any new developments, the president chose to downplay any of the risks associated with the approaching storm.

On January 20, 2020, the first case of coronavirus in the United States was reported in Washington State: a thirty-five-year-old man who had recently returned to the United States from Wuhan, China. In a television interview, the president was upbeat and reassuring to his audience: "We have it totally under control. It's one person coming from China, and we have it under control. It's going to be just fine." By January 30, there were five cases reported within the United States. Once again, the president was upbeat. Speaking at a campaign rally in Iowa, the president said, "We only have five people. Hopefully, everything's going to be great."[12]

On February 3, the CDC warned that we could expect to see many more cases. On February 10 and 11, the president reassured us some more: "Looks like by April, you know, in theory, when it gets a little warmer, it miraculously goes away. I hope that's true. But we're doing great in our country." The next day, with 12 cases having been reported in the United States, he reassured us that "in our country, we only have, basically, 12 cases and most of those people are recovering and some cases fully recovered. So, it's actually less." Then we had 15 cases. "When you have 15 people, and the 15 within a couple of days is going to be down to close to zero, that's a pretty good job we've done." By February 28, the United States had 60 cases, and experts were warning there would be many more. The president said, "Now the Democrats are politicizing the coronavirus . . . and this is their new hoax." By March 5, there were 217 U.S. cases and 12 American deaths. The president informed us that things were still great and that he was doing a great job: "Gallup just gave us the highest rating ever for the way we are handling the coronavirus situation." A few days later, as the death toll increased to 28, we were told, "This was unexpected. . . . And it hit the world. And we're prepared, and we're doing a great job with it. And it will go away. Just stay calm. It will go away."

As these quotes might suggest, the messaging of the president seemed to contradict what the experts, including his own in the federal government, were saying. All of these perplexing quotes from the president as a global public health crisis reached our shores give rise to some questions that need to be answered. Why was the president playing down the threat of the COVID-19 pandemic? What exactly was he and his administration doing as the threat mounted? Were we responding as we needed to and in a timely manner?

To begin with, 2020 was an election year, and President Trump faced an uphill battle in his quest to win a second term. Trump's reflex is always to try to talk his way out of or around anything that might be damaging to his image and his political standing. Facts are not nearly so important as the impression he wishes to make. In this context, his statements about the approaching pandemic and its threats must be considered to be political damage control as opposed to public health advice. He was especially worried about the potential impact of a pandemic on the economy. The economy, which he felt was his strong suit in the coming election, needed to be reassured by a relentless assertion that the disease had been "contained" and that everything was "under control."

Larry Kudlow, chairman of the National Economic Council, eagerly enlisted in the cause. On February 25, he appeared on American television screens to assert, "We have contained this. I won't say it's airtight, but it's pretty close to airtight."[13] As these incredible words were leaving his lips, most people who had a clue about what was about to unfold as the virus spread across the nation were no doubt concerned about what this sort of ill-informed judgment might mean about the nation's preparedness to deal with what was actually coming. This comment by Mr. Kudlow and the president's constant downplaying of the threat were no doubt designed to encourage the stock market. The market was President Trump's primary barometer with respect to the economy, perhaps suggesting how little he really understood the complexities of the economy. Unfortunately, market reactions to the assertions of the president and others that things were "contained" were, on the whole, negative. Nevertheless, the electoral interests of Donald Trump would guide his response to the crisis from beginning to end.

More troublesome than the messaging and downplaying of the threat were the details about what was or was not actually being done at the federal level as the pandemic reached our shores. The administration's rosy messaging was fundamentally at odds with the reality of the situation. Alarm bells inside and outside of the U.S. government should have been sounding loudly. Public health officials the world over had warned as early as January that the unique features of this flu-like coronavirus made it impossible to control. Given everything that the experts were telling it, the administration should have used any time that containment measures might buy to prepare the country for an inevitable and serious outbreak.[14] The emphasis on denying visas to travelers from China, and later from Europe, and suggesting that this would keep the virus out of the United States was both misleading and tragically wrong. This "containment" policy was a Hail Mary doomed to fail. At best, it might buy some time to better prepare for the serious wave that was coming. The Trump administration's focus on this strategy and its public denial of the seriousness of the threat only succeeded in diverting attention and resources from the more important priorities related to mitigation and treatment.

When the outbreak finally hit with its full force, the administration was both behind and painfully slow to catch up. Testing for the new virus was an essential priority to be met. But in addition to not having enough testing kits available, those that had been secured proved to be faulty. This meant that vital information about the spread of the disease was not available in the early weeks of the crisis. Equally concerning, there were shortages of vital equipment needed by hospitals and public health departments to treat patients. As the United States stumbled out of the gate in dealing with the arrival of the virus to its shores, it was apparent to expert and nonexpert alike that the U.S. response was weeks, perhaps months, behind schedule.[15]

The initial efforts at containment, the closing of the United States to travelers from China and later Europe, were not wrong steps to take. They were meant to slow the spread and give us time to prepare. There was never any hope of keeping the virus out of the United States. In fact, it was already within U.S. borders and doing what all viruses do—spreading. Everything that was about to happen was predictable, and the Trump administration was making decisions that every expert was telling it would be ineffective and insufficient. Directing public health departments to focus all their attention on monitoring a small number of quarantined travelers returning to the United States only ensured that they would not be fully engaged in the more vital work needed to prepare mitigation efforts in their communities. The virus was already infecting more people than was being reported.

The things not being done were critical to understand. Health care workers should have been coordinating with hospitals. Efforts to track suspected cases, to prepare vulnerable populations for what was coming, and to communicate with the public to provide necessary reassurance and guidance should have been priorities. Instead, the administration operated on the assumption that such things were not necessary because the containment strategy would not fail. The message coming from our national leadership (contrary to all the evidence) was that "we are stopping this at our border." The repeated presidential assertions that the containment strategy was a success no doubt diminished the sense of urgency and, according to public health experts, caused delays in community preparedness across the nation.[16]

In an ideal situation, as the travel restrictions were being implemented, the federal government should have also focused on mobilizing the country for the outbreak of the pandemic within the United States. This meant improving the capacity to test for COVID-19 in anticipation of the first reported cases on U.S. soil, which would require sending test kits to hospitals and clinics around the nation to identify any new infections. Federal and state officials should have prepared for a rapid response. This would have included issuing public recommendations on sanitation practices and when to seek medical treatment and information about the necessary and effective defensive measures that should be taken to limit the spread of the disease.

The U.S. failure to quickly ramp up a response strategy and its delay in preparing the nation and its communities for what was coming had very serious repercussions. This failure exacerbated the spread of the disease, robbed public health officials of vital data about the spread of the virus, and slowed the nation's capacity to respond to an outbreak. As the coronavirus spread from Asia to Europe, Latin America, sub-Saharan Africa, and North America, the federal government's tardy response and its misleading and optimistic statements were conscious decisions that ignored both the reality of what was happening and the expert advice to accelerate preparations for mitigating and responding to a serious outbreak. Even as the first wave began to spread across the country—and oblivious to the fact that the low number of reported cases was primarily due to the fact that very few people were being tested—the administration continued to claim that the containment strategy was working. The president insisted that the media and Democrats were exaggerating the threat in an effort to inflict political damage on him in an election year. At a February 27 press conference, the president said, "We have had tremendous success, tremendous success, beyond what people would have thought."[17]

By mid-January to late January, it was clear to most public health experts that a major public health crisis was unavoidable. It was clear that keeping the virus out of the country was a pipe dream. The federal government should have been giving state and local governments as well as the American public an accurate description of what was to be expected. The emphasis should have been on taking the steps necessary to prepare for a major outbreak of the coronavirus. It was already in the country, and its spread could not be avoided. Steps taken to slow that spread, to plan for an increased caseload, to assist hospitals and health providers to scale up and be equipped, and to alert all to the probability of various defensive measures (social distancing, hygiene measures, possible closures, etc.) would have been in order. Instead, the federal government told us that containment had been "a tremendous success." As a result, as state after state began to experience the "wave," they were each left pretty much on their own to figure things out. Thankfully, some did. Unfortunately, some did not quite figure it out. In the absence of national guidance and a coherent national strategy, the state-by-state response was a scattershot approach that was less than ideal. Instead of a national strategy, the United States seemed at times to be running in fifty different directions.

By the end of May, one hundred thousand Americans had died from the COVID-19 outbreak. In just over four months, the United States became the global hot spot for the pandemic. With more confirmed cases than any other nation, the "tremendous success" in containing the virus that our president had repeatedly boasted about had proven to be a mirage. Perhaps it would be more accurate to say it had always been a presidential self-delusion.

Before examining the response of state leaders to the spread of the virus, a quick summary of the confusing strategy and the mixed messaging of the federal government is in order. The picture that emerges makes two things very clear. First, President Bush was absolutely correct in 2005 when, in response to the H5N1 scare and the acceleration of concerns about pandemic preparedness, he said, "We need a national strategy." Second, as events unfolded during the COVID-19 pandemic, we did not have a national strategy. All the good work of the two preceding administrations to develop such a strategy was of no avail as the United States stumbled along and struggled to deal with the reality of a global pandemic. There was nothing resembling a coherent national response to guide states and localities, and there was a good deal of confusion, as the messaging was repeatedly contradicted by the day-to-day events that unfolded. The time line from January through April shows a federal government reacting (too slowly) as opposed to staying ahead of developments.[18] It shows a woefully unprepared response that produced as much confusion as constructive action. After the first four months, with 100,000 Americans dead, 1.7 million cases, and forty million Americans unemployed, "tremendous success" was not exactly the phrase to best describe the American response efforts.

The Governors Respond: Inconsistency Reigns

The state-by-state response to the COVID-19 outbreak was seriously handicapped by the lack of coherent and consistent guidance from the federal government. It was handicapped even more by the slowness of the federal government to see any need to be proactive. During the early weeks of 2020, while President Trump assured everyone that "the coronavirus is very much under control," the things that the federal government was not doing mattered most of all. It was during these critical early weeks and months that the United States should have been stockpiling protective gear for health care providers and frontline workers. The national stockpile of N95 protective masks, gowns, and other supplies was woefully inadequate after years of underfunding. The federal government should have also accelerated activities to make testing widely available. Other countries were more proactive and efficient in accomplishing this. In South Korea, a country whose first confirmed case of COVID-19 coincided with that of the United States, the national government bought 720,000 masks for employees of businesses considered at risk of exposure to the coronavirus. When asked whether the U.S. federal government would supply personal protective equipment (PPE) from the national stockpile to states, President Trump responded that he would not act as a "shipping clerk."[19] At the outset, the states were left entirely on their own to acquire the needed PPE and other materials and were often in competition with each other for the limited supplies available in the marketplace.

It was especially troublesome that the United States did a poor job of scaling up testing for the coronavirus. As a comparative measure, consider how long it took the United States to reach one test per one thousand residents after it had reached the milestone of one thousand confirmed cases. Compared to other nations, the United States was dreadfully slow to hit that mark. It took Iceland only one day to reach a daily testing rate of one test per one thousand residents after surpassing the milestones of one thousand total confirmed cases and at least one hundred cases per million residents. It took Lithuania, Norway, and New Zealand seven, eight, and fourteen days, respectively, to reach that same daily testing rate. It took the United States fifty-five days to reach that same rate. The Trump administration more or less dragged its feet for nearly two months while millions of Americans were exposed to the virus before reliable testing became available.[20] Even then, it was never made available in sufficient quantities to keep pace with a rapidly growing need for testing.

In March, as states began to report shortages of medical equipment, including ventilators and face masks, federal assistance was slow and insufficient. The U.S. Department of Health and Human Services had requested $2 billion for additional medical equipment in February, but the White House only agreed to finance $500,000's worth. From the very beginning, advice from federal agencies was plagued by inconsistencies. The CDC, for example, was inconsistent in its face mask recommendations. This undoubtedly reflected the state of the science to some extent. It would be April before enough research confirmed the effectiveness of face masks in slowing or preventing the spread of the disease. After initially telling people that face masks were not necessary, the agency reversed course as the science on the matter became more solid. One also suspects the deemphasizing of face masks during the first months was to preserve the limited supply of surgical masks for health care providers who would soon be overwhelmed with the need for them. To complicate things further, states followed a piecemeal approach, with some requiring face masks and others not recommending them at all. What was needed was strong federal leadership and guidance. Absent that leadership, what was left was a confusing array of policies from the different states that were not necessarily being guided by the best public health expertise and scientific principles.[21]

As any pandemic emerges, the most critical concerns center around the fact that there is no vaccine for it and often no effective treatment measures. Because it is a new virus, it is likely that there are no antivirals or effective treatment options available. The only weapon to address the unfolding public health threat is the implementation of appropriate defensive measures. This means informing the public about the importance and effectiveness of social distancing measures and hygiene practices that can slow the spread of the virus. Inevitably, it will also likely mean a number of other things. These include the quick ramping up of testing capacity in hot spots, restrictions on social gatherings, the quarantine of infected persons, the closing of schools and businesses, and, ultimately, the implementation of stay-at-home orders. Each of these defensive measures are a part of a necessary effort to "flatten the curve" of infection (i.e., slow the spread of the disease). This is necessary to prevent hospitals and medical facilities from being overrun and to ensure that all who are infected may receive medical treatment.

In anticipation of a shortage of supplies, insufficient space in emergency rooms, and expected staff shortages at the onset of any pandemic, the implementation of defensive measures is the best initial step to be taken in response to a pandemic. But these defensive measures must be taken in a timely manner, and each step taken must be driven by scientific and public health considerations. Taking them too late, imperfectly implementing them, or ending them too early may make these defensive measures less effective than they ideally should be in the middle of a pandemic. As COVID-19 began its spread across the United States, and absent any definitive federal guidelines, states and localities had to make these sorts of decisions on the run. State governors in particular were critical decision makers as the virus made its inexorable and tragic cross-country journey.

On March 19, California Governor Gavin Newsom, in response to the rapidly growing number of coronavirus cases in his state, issued the first statewide stay-at-home order. New York Governor Andrew Cuomo did the same on March 20. New York City was quickly becoming the epicenter for COVID-19 in the United States. The first case of community spread had been reported in New Rochelle, a suburb of New York City, on March 2. By March 2, there were 216 confirmed cases in the state. That number rose to 613 by March 14 and would continue to rise. By late May, there were over 74,000 cases of coronavirus in the United States. About half of those cases, almost ten times more than any other state, were in New York City. Given the density of New York City (over 27,000 people per square mile), the number of international travelers arriving in the city each day, and the crowded conditions of city life, it made sense that New York City would become the first U.S. epicenter for the pandemic. Many would in fact argue that, despite their aggressive action, Governor Cuomo and New York City Mayor Bill de Blasio were slow when it came to taking the most aggressive measures that were needed and ultimately taken. In other words, they reacted to events rather than anticipating them. Yet, they would soon act with urgency and with considerable effectiveness.[22]

Governor Cuomo and Mayor de Blasio did limit public gatherings of over five hundred people in the city on March 12. As the virus continued to rapidly spread, that would lead to a more aggressive response. In contrast, and in anticipation of what was to come, California moved more quickly in taking aggressive measures to limit social life. The City of San Francisco issued a shelter-in-place order on March 12, and on March 19, with nine hundred cases statewide, Governor Newsom issued a statewide stay-at-home order. It is important to remember that the imposing of such restrictions, as difficult and as unpopular as they may be, cannot be done too early in a pandemic scenario. Just a few days can make a huge difference in containing the spread of the virus. One of the most positive things New York's governor had done early on was to quickly ramp up testing. The United States was lagging far behind most other countries in testing, but New York made a dedicated push to speed up testing at hospitals, labs, and drive-through centers set up in the most densely populated areas. It even pursued and received FDA approval to set up twenty-eight public and private labs for testing. This was done on March 13, making New York the first state to do so.[23]

It is safe to say that the nation was riveted to the scenes on their televisions coming out of New York City. The overcrowding of hospitals and intensive care units, the growing number of dead bodies (many stored in refrigerated trucks), the overworked medical staffs (hailed as heroes), and the haunting visions of the total shutdown of New York City left an impression on the nation. Governor Cuomo and Mayor de Blasio did, after what some felt was a slow start, take the aggressive actions needed to flatten the curve. They emphasized that their decisions were driven by the science and data and that public health was their sole focus. Soon, Governor Cuomo's daily press briefings became must-see TV, and the cable channels aired them in their entirety. His focus on the facts, the science if you will, and his compelling explanations of what was being done and why it was being done may have been the first coherent and effective explanation of the pandemic that many Americans had heard. The governor of New York was perceived by many as filling a leadership gap and making the crisis intelligible to the nation.

Still, it would seem that many citizens living in other parts of the country (and their governors and other elected officials) thought this was a New York problem. Many people in other parts of the country believed the pandemic would not impact them as badly as it had New York. Competent and informed leadership would have told them to be prepared. Cities, towns, and counties all across the country had to be told to expect the unwelcomed coronavirus to visit them with similar intensity in due time. New York should have been the ringing of an alarm bell warning other states and communities to prepare. Some heard and responded to the alarm; some did not. In just a couple of short weeks, we would see how other parts of the country were responding.

President Donald Trump, it might be argued, was not up to the task of providing the sort of leadership the crisis required. One can debate whether he was unwilling or unable to do so, but the result was that he did not play the part of a national leader. He did not unify the nation, and he did not take the sort of decisive action required to respond to a global pandemic. It would soon become apparent that the leadership needed during a public health crisis would have to come, if it came at all, from state executives throughout the nation. Not surprising, perhaps, politics would play a role in how governors across the nation responded to the challenge. Most Democratic governors emphasized the science of the matter and were willing to take more aggressive steps to slow the spread of the coronavirus. For most of them, it was a public health emergency to be addressed above all else. Many Republican governors emphasized the themes of the president (e.g., "everything's under control") and prioritized keeping the economy open. For them, the disaster would be to close things down and harm the strong economy that was the supposed key to the electoral success of the president and the Republican Party in November. There were, of course, exceptions to this generalization, but things did play out pretty much along partisan lines.

California's Democratic governor, Gavin Newsom, was the first governor to issue a statewide order to shutter businesses and keep people at home. Three days earlier, public health officials in six Bay Area counties had gone first and issued a joint stay-at-home order. This strong and timely action did seem to bend the curve, or slow the spread, as intended. California's number of COVID-19 confirmed cases and deaths rose more slowly than in the hard-hit states such as New York, New Jersey, Louisiana, and Michigan. This early success would not preclude later spikes in infections as things opened back up, but it was considered essential to controlling the outbreak at its beginning.[24]

One Republican governor who had the right priorities and acted decisively was Ohio's Mike DeWine. Even before Ohio had experienced its first outbreak of COVID-19, DeWine was the nation's first governor to call for the statewide closure of public schools. He also delayed the state's primary elections, snubbing an initial court order challenging his authority to do so that was constitutionally dubious. He was, above all else, data-driven in his decision-making. He implemented a timely stay-at-home order and was generally credited with calm but firm leadership that significantly slowed the spread of the virus. He was not in the least interested in taking his lead from President Trump and was more than willing to defy presidential edicts and whims. When the president tried to set the national goal for reopening the economy by Easter, DeWine pushed back, saying, "When people are dying, when people don't feel safe, the economy is not gonna come back."[25]

The state of Washington identified the first American case of COVID-19 and suffered the nation's first cluster of nursing home deaths. After being shown data in early March that argued for aggressive social distancing, Democratic Governor James Inslee immediately moved to ban large gatherings and prepared the public for more stringent measures. His quick and decisive action, taken early, seemed to pay off, as Washington's curve of coronavirus deaths flattened faster than any other state. Inslee was the first, but certainly not the last, governor to spar with the president over the pandemic response. On February 27, he met with Vice President Mike Pence to discuss the coronavirus outbreak. They had a rather pointed exchange during which Inslee said to the press afterward, "I told him our work would be more successful if the Trump administration stuck to the science and told the truth." The president responded with insults, calling Inslee a "snake," and publicly encouraged Pence not to call him anymore.[26]

Another Republican governor who acted aggressively to contain the spread of the virus was Maryland's Larry Hogan. In addition to timely and aggressive social distancing policies, Governor Hogan was quite willing to publicly disagree with the president. In a cable television interview, he was asked whether Maryland's social distancing policies matched Trump's suggestion that it would soon be time to ease up on such measures. Governor Hogan pointedly said, "They don't really match. Quite frankly, some of the messaging is pretty confusing. And I think it's not just that it doesn't match with what we're doing here in Maryland; some of the messaging coming out of the administration doesn't match." Hogan also coauthored a bipartisan *Washington Post* op-ed with Michigan's Democratic Governor Gretchen Whitmer that listed all the ways Washington and the federal government had not sufficiently helped the nation's governors.[27]

Ron DeSantis, Florida's Republican governor, was among the slowest in the nation to respond to COVID-19. He refused to shut down Florida's beaches as they were overrun with partiers during spring break. There was no doubt that the arrival of so many young people from all parts of the nation would increase the spread of the virus in Florida. DeSantis also stubbornly refused to issue a statewide stay-at-home order, at least until it was much too late in the game. He justified this by saying, "We're also in a situation where we have counties who have no community spread." He added, "We have some counties that don't have a single positive test yet." Of course, everything that the experts know about pandemics suggests you do not want to wait until you have community spread before taking strong action.[28] Governor DeSantis repeatedly emphasized that social distancing measures were too harmful to the economy. This was the message embraced by President Trump and echoed by a number of other Republican governors. Mississippi's Republican governor resisted a statewide stay-at-home order on ideological grounds, insisting that "Mississippi's never going to be China. Mississippi's never going to be North Korea." A rising infection rate would eventually drag him into issuing such an order, but it would not be as extensive or as successful as it might have been due to its broadly defining what business and social activities were considered to be "essential"—including religious services.[29]

Alabama's Kay Ivey, another Republican governor who refused to issue a timely stay-at-home order, was persistent in her refusal to address the public health crisis with an aggressive response. As Alabama's caseload grew, she responded by observing, "Y'all, we are not Louisiana, we are not New York State, we are not California." Her own lieutenant governor, Republican Will Ainsworth, found her response to be inadequate. He served on Governor Ivey's coronavirus task force. On March 25, discouraged by the weak response that was unfolding in Alabama, he wrote a letter to the other members of the task force in which he stated, "A tsunami of hospital patients is likely to fall upon Alabama in the not-too-distant future, and it is my opinion that this task force and the state are not taking a realistic view of the numbers or adequately preparing for what awaits us." Frankly, this same message could have justifiably been sent to many Republican governors across the country.[30]

Following the lead of President Trump in downplaying the threat, defining the choices to be made as binary (i.e., one must choose between the economy or public health), and being deaf to the scientific expertise, these governors resisted the social distancing and other measures that were proven to be the best options for slowing the spread of the virus. Most would, reluctantly and much too late, eventually implement such measures, but they would also relax them too quickly. Because solving the public health emergency was not their first priority, mainly because they thought the economic consequences of making it such were unacceptable, these governors only succeeded in guaranteeing that the public health consequences for their states and their citizens would become more severe. The science, if they had paid any attention to it, would have told them that things would get worse. It was only a matter of time. Ironically, their resistance to the science had severe economic consequences as well.

Someone with a reasonable understanding of pandemic scenarios would have been able to make reasonable predictions about what would follow in the months ahead based on observations of the patchwork of state-by-state responses during the first four months of 2020. COVID-19 would not be under control. Its first wave would not end, as the states that had been in denial about the need to act aggressively and were slow to respond would reap the consequences of their delay or inaction. Any person with a reasonable understanding of the COVID-19 pandemic would have known that states such as Florida, Mississippi, Alabama, South Carolina, and Texas would become raging hot spots for new infections. But truth be told, it was not just the Republican governors who were not taking the pandemic seriously. They were aided and abetted by citizens who also did not take the pandemic seriously. Given the conflicting messages they were receiving and the chaotic confusion of national, state, and local response efforts, it is perhaps understandable that some citizens were not taking things as seriously as one might have hoped. Also, and most unfortunately, just as there was a partisan divide among the nation's governors with respect to their response to the public health emergency, partisan division was also one of the factors in the public response.

The Public Response

How did the American public respond during the first wave of the COVID-19 pandemic? Very early on, one was apt to hear some citizens opine, "I don't think it will be all that bad." Perhaps the assumption was that this is the United States, and we are better prepared than most countries to deal with issues of public health. As the number of coronavirus cases began to surge in many states across the country, citizens began to show some healthy concern for their health and safety. They most certainly worried about the possibility of catching the new disease. They also worried about ending up in the hospital and, worse, in intensive care. They began to show concern for the ways in which the disease might spread and seemed willing to undertake reasonable hygiene and social distancing precautions. Some were no doubt oblivious to these concerns, but public opinion surveys did show a growing level of public concern in the spring of 2020.

By late April, COVID-19 was a matter of intense concern for most Americans. By the end of June, the level of concern seemed to be in decline (see table 4.1). As the summer wore on and spikes in infections increased across parts of the nation, the level of concern rose again. As one might expect, the level of personal concern about the virus varied and would continue to vary significantly across demographic groups. This is a reflection of their differing risk factors and, not surprisingly,

Table 4.1 Concerns over Health Impacts of COVID-19

Percent who say they are very or somewhat concerned that they might get COVID and require hospitalization

	April	June
Total	55%	51%
Republican	47%	35%
Democrat	64%	62%
White	51%	43%
Black	63%	59%
Hispanic	73%	70%

Percent who say they are concerned that they might unknowingly spread COVID-19 to others

	April	June
Total	62%	66%
Republican	58%	45%
Democrat	74%	77%
White	56%	65%
Black	64%	72%
Hispanic	75%	79%

Source: Pew Research Center, June 25, 2020, https://www.pewresearch.org/politics /2020/06/25/republicans-democrats-move-even-further-apart-in-coronavirus -concerns/

their differing partisan perspectives. Because these variations were to be expected, it once again emphasizes the critical importance of clear and accurate messaging by leaders to pull the nation together.

The concern about the health impacts of COVID-19 and the spread of the virus were consistently higher among Democrats than among Republicans. In early April, a 58 percent majority of Republicans said they were concerned they may spread the disease without knowing it, and nearly half (47 percent) were concerned they would get a serious case of COVID-19. At that same time, 64 percent of Democrats were concerned that they might be infected, and 74 percent were concerned they may spread the disease without knowing it. Among the public as a whole, health concerns from the coronavirus changed little in the two-month period between April and the end of June. But the partisan divide as well as the racial and ethnic differences in concerns about unknowingly spreading COVID-19 or contracting a serious case of the disease widened. Republican concerns had lessened over that two-month period, while Democrat concerns remained steady. Notably, concerns over unknowingly spreading the coronavirus increased 8 percentage points among Black Americans (from 64 percent to 72 percent) between April and June while decreasing by about the same amount (from 65 percent to 56 percent) among white Americans. This may reflect the fact that Black Americans were generally found to be at higher risk for more severe impacts if infected. It may also reflect the fact that Republicans are predominantly white, and as their "concerns" lessened, it accentuated the differences along racial lines. The June Pew Research Center poll also found that six in ten U.S. adults (59 percent) believed that ordinary Americans have a great deal of impact on the spread of the coronavirus. But here also the partisan differences were significant. While 73 percent of Democrats thought the actions of ordinary people mattered a great deal in affecting its spread, only 44 percent of Republicans said the same.[31]

By April, the number of states that had issued stay-at-home orders gave rise to an interesting question. How would Americans feel about complying with such orders? From mid-March to mid-April, Gallup tracked the willingness of Americans to comply with requests by public health officials for people to remain home in the event of a serious coronavirus outbreak in their community (see table 4.2). It was during this time period that such requests were being made because cases were spiking in various parts of the country. Throughout the one-month period, Gallup found no more than 67 percent of U.S. adults said they were very likely to comply. The number varied over the month. In mid-March, 41 percent said they were very likely to comply. This number would increase to 67 percent from March 30 to April 5. This increase occurred as nearly every state had issued, or begun to issue, stay-at-home orders. By the end of April, there was a slight decline, with 62 percent saying they were likely to comply.

Partisan differences were, not unexpectedly, observable. Support for compliance did increase among all partisan groups at the beginning of data collection. Over time, the support for stay-at-home orders among Democrats remained near its peak, whereas support among Republicans and independents declined somewhat.[32] The slight decline observed in support for stay-at-home orders occurred as groups of protesters across the country started to pressure leaders to reopen the economy. This was something to be expected perhaps. But support for the stay-at-home orders remained high, as the protesters represented a very small minority. Table 4.2 shows what the support looked like at the end of April.

At the end of April, polling consistently showed that Americans supported the stay-at-home orders. They also did not want to fully reopen too

Table 4.2 Americans' Likelihood to Comply with Stay-at-Home Orders

If public health officials recommended that everyone stay at home for a month because of a serious outbreak of coronavirus, how likely are you to stay home for a month?

	Very Likely	Somewhat Likely	Somewhat Unlikely	Very Unlikely
All	62%	19%	8%	11%
Democrats	76%	----	----	----
Republicans	47%	----	----	----
Independents	56%	----	----	----
Age 18–44	63%	----	----	----
Age 45–64	57%	----	----	-----
Age 65 and over	70%	----	----	-----

Source: Gallup, https://news.gallup.com/opinion/gallup/309491/compliance-curve -americans-stay-home-covid.aspx

quickly because they perceived a serious health risk from doing so. The worry about reopening was perhaps the most interesting finding. A Pew Research Center poll asked, "Thinking about the decisions by a number of state governments to impose significant restrictions on public activity because of the coronavirus outbreak, is your greater concern that state governments will lift the restrictions too quickly or not quickly enough?" Among all respondents, 66 percent said they worried about lifting the restrictions too quickly, while 32 percent said they worried about not lifting the restrictions quickly enough. Among Democrats, 81 percent said they worried more about lifting restrictions too quickly, while among Republicans, 51 percent said so.[33] A Yahoo News–YouGov poll released April 20 asked, "In considering whether to reopen the economy, are you more concerned about lifting the restrictions too quickly or too slowly?" Among all respondents, 71 percent said they were more concerned about the restrictions being lifted too quickly. The partisan divide on this question was 85 percent for Democrats and 56 percent for Republicans. An NBC News–Wall Street Journal poll released on April 20 asked, "Which worries you more . . . that the United States will move too quickly in loosening restrictions and the virus will continue to spread with more lives being lost, or that the United States will take too long in loosening restrictions and the economic impact will be even worse with more jobs being lost?" Overall, 58 percent said they worried more about lifting the restrictions too soon.[34]

At the end of April, it can be concluded that a large majority of Americans, and even a sizable majority of Republicans, remained concerned that lifting stay-at-home orders could result in an accelerated spread of coronavirus. Between 58 percent and 81 percent of Americans were supportive of keeping the stay-at-home restrictions in place for the time being or even expanding them to the nation as a whole. In fact, a Quinnipiac poll found that 81 percent of the respondents said they supported a national order. The idea garnered support from 95 percent of Democrats, 68 percent of Republicans, and 80 percent of independents.[35]

While it was encouraging to see that public concern about the spread of the virus and support for stay-at-home orders were both very high, this did not mean that people would not tire quickly of such restrictions. Neither did it mean that those in the minority would remain quiet or that there would be no controversy. On April 22, the United States reported the highest single-day death toll (2,600) recorded by any nation up to that time. In the next four weeks, the U.S. death toll would reach 91,938. By May 20, the United States had recorded 1,528,661 reported cases of COVID-19. These numbers would only continue to increase. By July 12, the United States had reached 3,366,515 confirmed cases and 137,191 deaths. Worldwide, on that same date, there were 12,768,307 confirmed cases and 566,654 COVID deaths in 216 countries or territories.[36] These case numbers and the rising death toll suggest, at the very least, that it was quite rational for Americans in April to support the stay-at-home orders and to worry about the safety of opening their states back up. But the political dynamic in the United States would have a much greater impact on what was to follow than the consensus in favor of the restrictions and the perceived need for caution.

To begin with, the U.S. stay-at-home orders were not national policy. They were implemented state by state in a piecemeal fashion and typically after a major outbreak of the virus (that should have been anticipated) was already upon them. This contrasted dramatically with the European responses to the pandemic. European nations reacted with a national approach as opposed to piecemeal regional or local responses. Their shutdowns were, in many cases, more timely and more thorough than the American response. This helped them to "flatten the curve" and reduce the spread of the virus a bit more efficiently than the United States would be able to do. Some U.S. governors, as we have seen, were either slow to act or resistant to the need to act, and the president of the United States was sending a different message with each passing day. He was initially resistant to state stay-at-home orders, then briefly supported them, and then quickly reversed course yet again to accuse governors (especially

Democratic governors) of going too far. For example, when asked whether he believed states such as Michigan, Minnesota, and Virginia should lift their stay-at-home orders, the president said, "I think elements of what they've done are too much, just too much. . . . What they've done in Virginia is just incredible."[37] This statement, uttered on April 17, was in the context of President Trump's insistence that the economy should be fully reopened by Easter.

Whether it was cues taken from the president or the growing uncertainty and fear over the economic impact of stay-at-home orders, in late April, there exploded onto the scene what one might call a culture war that pitted conservatives against liberals and the different regions of the country against each other. Conservatives, who tend to reside in rural areas, which were less impacted by the virus, generally opposed the stay-at-home orders, while liberals who resided in the urban areas most severely impacted by the virus generally supported them.

In several Midwestern states, and later in other parts of the country, protests broke out. Some protesters carried guns. Some waved Trump 2020 signs, and Confederate flags were a common sight. These protesters sought to frame the debate as a defense of constitutional freedoms. They saw stay-at-home orders and other restrictions states had introduced as excessive governmental overreach and an infringement on their liberty. These protesters were, as one would not be surprised to observe, egged on by conservative media and the president of the United States.

Michigan was a prime example of what was appearing on television screens across the country. The state had taken very big hits in both coronavirus cases and job losses. A movement called "Operation Gridlock" by its organizers held a demonstration against the strict stay-at-home policies ordered by Michigan's Democratic governor, Gretchen Whitmer. The demonstrators included members of far-right groups who had been a large presence at various pro-Trump and gun rights rallies across the state of Michigan. The demonstration peaked with armed protesters occupying the Michigan State Capitol. In what was becoming a regular routine, these protests were cheered on by conservative media.

Another regular part of the routine included President Trump posting highly incendiary tweets stoking angry protests against physical distancing requirements and other coronavirus stay-at-home measures in states led by Democratic governors. "LIBERATE MINNESOTA!" the U.S. president tweeted in capital letters. "LIBERATE MICHIGAN!" "LIBERATE VIRGINIA, and save your great 2nd Amendment. It is under siege!" This latter tweet was a reference to Virginia's Democratic governor, Ralph Northam, who had just signed into law new measures on gun control.[38]

It was inevitable, perhaps, but the worst thing that could possibly have happened to thwart a successful American response to the pandemic had happened. It had become a political issue rather than a public health issue. At a time when national unity would be required to save lives, division and conflict spread faster than the virus itself. When national leadership needed to work overtime to provide consistent messaging and promote unity, it produced conflicting messaging and fueled partisan division. To make matters even worse, the United States also struggled to get a handle on and manage the economic impacts of the pandemic. By the end of April, just four months into our disjointed and piecemeal response to COVID-19, there was reason to fear that the months to come would be very difficult in the United States.

The Economic Impacts of COVID-19

Inevitably, the implementation of public health measures and decisions to shut down public places or issue stay-at-home orders severed the flow of goods and people, stalled economies, and delivered a global recession. The economic contagion would spread with the virus and be severe in its impact on the global economy. With people unable to work, the supply chain would be weakened, if not broken.

As COVID-19 intensified, bringing thousands and then tens of thousands into the health care system, it also became necessary to shut down the economy. Social distancing and stay-at-home orders, which were necessary as a public health strategy to slow the spread of the virus, meant that governments discouraged and then prohibited people from going to work. What we collectively and unavoidably produced was a sudden contraction of the labor supply and a loss of employment and income for millions of Americans. Between mid-March and mid-April, twenty-two million Americans filed for unemployment benefits. By the end of May, forty million Americans had filed for unemployment. This was a nearly 15 percent unemployment rate compared to the 3.5 percent rate in early March.[39] While some analysts suggested that these unemployment numbers would bounce back quickly when the threat of the virus had been contained and the economy reopened, others pointed out that many businesses would never reopen. Instead of a quick recovery and a return to normal, they warned of a long and difficult road ahead. More immediately, millions of Americans were now without income in the middle of a pandemic. Needless to say, such dramatic unemployment numbers meant that policy makers would have to consider legislation to help mitigate the economic burden on families and businesses.

On March 18, Congress passed the Families First Coronavirus Act. This legislation provided $192 billion in federal money to enhance unemployment benefits, increase federal Medicaid and food security spending, and provide free coverage of coronavirus testing under government health programs. It also required certain employers to provide paid sick leave.[40] On March 27, Congress enacted the CARES Act. This was a relief package of around $2 trillion to address the near-term economic impact the virus was having on families and businesses. One of the key items in the legislation included $500 billion to be used to assist companies that are critical to national security and distressed sectors of the economy. Of that sum, about $450 billion was meant to support loans to businesses, states, and municipalities through a new Federal Reserve lending facility. Other items included economic support for small businesses, an expansion of unemployment benefits, and federal aid to hospitals and health care providers. About $290 billion was allocated to make direct payments to taxpayers. Taxpayers with annual incomes of up to $75,000 (or $150,000 for married couples) would receive onetime payments of $1,200 (that payment amount gradually phased out for high-income earners, with a cap at an annual salary of $99,000 or $198,000 for married couples). Families would also receive an additional $500 per qualifying child.[41]

An interesting part of the CARES Act was something called the Paycheck Protection Program (PPP). The federal government set aside $349 billion for the PPP. This program was run by the Small Business Administration (SBA), and an additional $310 billion was added to it in late April. Under this program, small businesses (i.e., those with fewer than five hundred employees) could take out loans to pay for workers' salaries, health care benefits, and sick leave as well as other key expenses, such as rent and utilities. People who were self-employed or working as independent contractors were also eligible to borrow through the PPP.

As wonderful as all of this sounds, there was great controversy surrounding the PPP, which had a lot to do with who benefited the most from the program. The stated goal of the PPP was to keep American workers on payroll, not to simply keep small businesses going. Even so, the program was widely perceived as being meant to boost the most vulnerable small businesses. In practice, however, it ended up prioritizing businesses that were not actually that small. Most of the loans were disbursed to businesses with more employees rather than to smaller businesses with fewer employees. Larger companies sucked up most of the loan money, and many small businesses never really had a chance for loan approval. According to the SBA, the average PPP loan was $107,000. If businesses spent 75 percent of the loan money on payroll, the loan would be forgivable within eight weeks. After receiving some feedback from the business community, Congress changed the parameters of the loans in mid-June to require 60 percent be spent on payroll over a period of twenty-four weeks. But small businesses were simply not being helped much at all.[42]

Minority-owned businesses, in particular, received little to no PPP assistance. Part of the reason for this was that many banks approving PPP loans only accepted applications from existing customers. Needless to say, that left out many minority-owned businesses that had weak relationships or no relationships at all with banks. Also, not surprisingly, because banks could collect bigger fees for bigger loans, they were further incentivized to prioritize bigger businesses over the smaller ones. The federal government would perhaps have been better advised to set up a system to give money directly to workers or to small businesses. Instead, the financial institutions did things as they normally do, which is to say they brought with them the flaws and biases of the private market.[43] This did not bode well for small businesses, which are considered the backbone of the American economy. The PPP was intended to help employers keep operations running despite revenue shortfalls. It basically failed to achieve that objective. Large, publicly traded companies received massive sums, while small businesses were in too many cases left frustrated and without help.

Despite all the legislation enacted by Congress, too many Americans received too little easing of the economic burdens inflicted by the pandemic. A onetime $1,200 check from Uncle Sam would not make much of a dent in the problem for most families. As unemployment rates increased, the number of applications for benefits overloaded the system and delayed the process of obtaining relief. The PPP seemed to provide more protection for the well-to-do and not nearly enough for small businesses and their employees. The programs enacted were quickly shown not to be enough as they ran out of money and the pandemic raged on. The economic struggles of families, the mounting threats to the survival of many small businesses, and the growing worries about job loss and lack of income undoubtedly contributed to the impatience and anger over stay-at-home orders and other restrictions, and they certainly contributed to a sense of urgency about taking whatever risks were involved with reopening the economy. There is also no doubt that a more effective and urgent response to the pandemic by our federal government would have reduced some of the economic impacts that had befallen the nation. However, that would have required a response driven by expertise—by science—not by politics. And that would have required a national strategy and the meeting of a very high bar for leadership. Indeed, the most important variable that may contribute to success in dealing with a public health emergency is the relationship between scientific expertise and political leadership. In 2020, that relationship in the United States was, in a word, inadequate for the COVID-19 challenge.

The President and the Experts: The War Within

As 2020 began with an exploding global public health crisis approaching the United States, each passing day made it more and more apparent to many experts that the U.S. federal government's response to COVID-19 was appallingly slow and inadequate. This should have surprised no one. President Donald Trump disliked and distrusted experts of all kinds. He especially had very little use for the career bureaucrats who actually make the government function. He had spent a good portion of his presidency attacking these kinds of nonpartisan career experts and professionals as a "swamp" that needed to be drained.

In part, the president's disdain for the professionals in government can be explained by his brand of populism. Donald Trump got elected by tapping into the populist sentiments of the kind found in Tea Party circles. The worldview that these conservative populists embrace is profoundly anti-elitist, anti-intellectual, and anti-government. The anger and resentment they feel as self-perceived victims of the elites and intellectuals was something that Trump manipulated most expertly. These conservative populists were a loyal base of support for Donald Trump, and he worked ceaselessly to play to them.

To the motivation of pleasing his political base can be added Donald Trump's own distrust, and even fear, of experts. Once in office, President Trump faced the thing he detested the most. He encountered, as he knew he would, resistance from bureaucratic experts in the government as he proceeded to break the norms of executive branch practices on issue after issue. His intolerance for any fact that disrupted his preferred narrative, his obsession with himself and his own imagined brilliance, his thirst for adulation, and no doubt his fear of his own inadequacies being uncovered required him to discredit and disparage the very bureaucratic experts who would so desperately be needed to guide us through something like a global pandemic. It was no surprise then when it was reported in April 2020 that President Trump had ignored experts on COVID-19 for months.[44]

From the beginning of January 2020, President Trump was seemingly disinterested as experts and administration officials tried to warn him about the serious nature of the coronavirus pandemic. He showed little interest in government authorities as they proposed strategies for dealing with the pandemic. Even as he restricted travel from China into the United States, the president played down the threat his experts and advisers were warning him about. He repeatedly told administration officials not to "panic" over COVID-19. Throughout January and February, the president received memos urging him to think about things such as social distancing, quarantining, and more intensive efforts aimed at pandemic preparedness. Even his trade adviser, Peter Navarro, was urging the president to take the threat of a global pandemic seriously.[45]

On February 24, the White House Coronavirus Task Force wanted to present to the president a plan for mitigation. This plan was a comprehensive strategy for containing the effects of the virus once it began to spread within the country. Among other things, it discussed and provided guidance for things such as school dismissals and cancellations of mass gatherings. It discussed the need and planned for aggressive testing, quarantining, and social distancing efforts. But the group never got to present the plan. Why? Because President Trump was infuriated over a CDC statement. The director of the CDC's National Center for Immunization and Respiratory Diseases announced in a press conference on February 26 that the virus was here and warned that it was spreading.[46] This was not a fact welcomed by the president nor one that he wanted to have widely reported. He was irate that his messaging that things were "under control" had been contradicted by a CDC expert. This is not exactly surprising news given Mr. Trump's history. The biggest take away from such reports is that many people within the administration, along with all the public health experts in our federal agencies, understood and correctly foresaw the need to act quickly and effectively to prepare for the pandemic. President Trump had had ample opportunity to take wise and more aggressive steps much earlier in response to a looming public health disaster. Instead, his delays and refusal to listen to experts led the country to a worst-case scenario that might have been avoided. At the very least, it may have saved many lives in the difficult months ahead.

It can be suggested that President Trump had impeded the nation's ability to effectively respond to the COVID-19 pandemic years before the outbreak in 2020. This is in reference to his decision to eliminate the body in the National Security Council that had been created during the Obama administration to be responsible for ongoing planning for public health emergencies, including pandemics. During his presidency, he had also eroded the CDC budget and autonomy. When the first pandemic wave hit the United States, the president compounded the crisis by allowing political concerns and infighting to take priority over swift and effective responsiveness. It was not a lack of expertise or a lack of ability to implement a workable strategy to combat the spread of COVID-19 that handicapped the U.S. response to COVID-19. It was the conscious actions and the decisions of a president to disregard the experts and ignore the threat that determined the design of everything that would follow.

From day one of his presidency, Donald Trump had declared war against science. His main objective was to weaken the influence of governmental scientists on public policy. The very moment he took the oath of office, all mention of climate change was removed from the White House web page. On day three, he barred employees of the Environmental Protection Agency (EPA) from posting updates on social media or providing information to reporters. The administration also mandated that all EPA studies first be reviewed and cleared by political staffers in the White House before being released to the public. In March 2017, the president proposed significant budget cuts for the EPA and CDC. A few months later, he officially withdrew the United States from the Paris climate accord.[47] His priorities were clear. The president sought to reduce the influence of science, reduce the ability of scientific agencies to communicate to the public, reduce budgets for these agencies, and eliminate as many governmental science-based regulations as possible.

This resistance to and, in many cases, denial of science were part of a broader effort. The goal was to tip the balance toward corporate and industrial interests in any area where science might impose unwelcomed doses of reality and suggest measures to promote things, such as public safety and health or environmental protection, that would slow down their trips to the bank with their profits. This is not to say that the administration was without the necessary expert talent and advice needed to orchestrate a more successful response to COVID-19 in 2020. All the weakening of the various scientific agencies and the abandoning of all the pandemic planning of the two previous administrations did not leave the administration unarmed in the face of a rapidly rising new threat. The administration simply consciously decided not to use the weapons at hand. Its response was not driven by science or by the experts.

Two of the experts merit special attention, as they would become very well known by the American public during the first six months of 2020. Both served on the White House Coronavirus Task Force and would become the voice of science (often resented or contradicted by the president) in the public briefings that were to follow. Dr. Anthony Fauci, director of the National Institute of Allergy and Infectious Diseases, was both impressively experienced and universally respected. He had advised six presidents on HIV/AIDS and many other domestic and global health issues. Fauci was one of the principal architects of the emergency health plan that provided AIDS relief throughout the developing world. This plan has been credited with saving millions of lives. The other expert, Dr. Deborah Birx, the U.S. global AIDS coordinator and U.S. special representative for health diplomacy, was equally impressive. In 1985, she began her work with the Department of Defense as a clinician in immunology who focused on HIV/AIDS vaccine research. From 2005 to 2014, she served as the director of the CDC's Division of Global HIV/AIDS. She also implemented the CDC's AIDS relief program that Dr. Fauci had helped design. These would be the two leading scientific experts most visible in the public arena occupied by the White House Coronavirus Task Force. That this task force was led by Vice President Pence rather than one of them might have been a hint that science would take a back seat to politics in the federal government's response to COVID-19.

Initially, the White House Coronavirus Task Force press briefings were conducted without the participation of President Trump. Typically, Vice President Pence began the briefing with some updates. These updates included long and gushy praise for the leadership of the president in his dealing with the crisis. Next, substantive and useful information was delivered by Drs. Fauci and Birx as well as other assorted experts. Soon President Trump was front and center in what became almost daily press briefings. One suspects his decision to take the lead at the briefings may have been motivated by the media praise New York Governor Cuomo was receiving for his data-driven and scientifically guided daily briefings. The typical performance by President Trump at his task force briefings was less impressive to many. Soon these briefings were being called "Trump's follies."

The typical briefing began with the president stumbling over written text he did not begin to understand. This was followed by his telling viewers what a great job he was doing. Next, a few experts or guests provided a little useful information and, in an embarrassing number of cases, lots of sappy praise for the president's leadership. The daily briefing than concluded with the president answering press queries by displaying his general ignorance and attacking the media. He often contradicted what the experts had just said.

The president's statements at the daily briefings always included ample self-praise: "I've felt it was a pandemic long before it was called a pandemic." He would tell us that even the experts were amazed at his insights. On March 6, he visited the CDC and used the occasion to remind us of just how smart he is: "Every one of these (CDC) doctors said, 'How do you know so much about this?' Maybe I have a natural ability. Maybe I should have done this instead of running for president." Back at the task force briefings, the president was asked what metrics he would use in deciding how and when to reopen the economy. The president pointed to his temple and said, "The metrics right here."

President Trump was very pleased with his performance at these briefings and proclaimed them to be a great success. Why? What was the basis for his claim of success? In a tweet on March 29, he said that success was measured by the ratings of his news conferences. He bragged that his ratings were "Bachelor-finale, Monday-Night-Football type of numbers." At the March 29 White House task force briefing, the president gave himself credit for the attention Governor Cuomo was receiving. He also said he had made stars of other people: "We're getting the accurate word out. And a lot of people aren't. But they should be happy. When I have the General, when I have Seema (Verma, head of Medicare and Medicaid Services), and when I have Tony (Fauci), and when I have our . . . our in— . . . our incred— . . . these are, like people that have become big stars, okay?"

Always on display during these briefings was the president's total lack of understanding of a pandemic. On April 10, when asked if reopening the country would depend on surveillance and contact tracing, the president replied such tests were not necessary because "vast areas of the country" did not have outbreaks.[48] In addition to being 100 percent wrong—in fact, every state had recorded coronavirus cases—it revealed his ignorance of the basics of the potential for exponential growth in the spread of a highly contagious virus.

The best indicator of President Trump's leadership failures during the first wave of the pandemic may be the number of times that medical experts found it necessary to push back against his statements and suggestions. The president found himself touting unproven treatments or misstating facts so often that experts had to contradict him on a regular basis. He had spent weeks pushing hydroxychloroquine, an antimalarial drug, as a "game changer" in the treatment of COVID-19. The Food and Drug Administration issued a statement on April 24 urging caution and bluntly stating, "Hydroxychloroquine and chloroquine have not been shown to be safe and effective for treating or preventing COVID-19." This was one of many instances in which the medical experts pushed back against the president's COVID-19 messaging.[49]

Many of President Trump's advisers were concerned that his rambling commentaries in the daily task force briefings were too long, too frequently devolving into unrelated political issues, too frequently degenerating into shouting matches with the assembled media, and too often a source of political controversy. They thought it might be time to end the president's daily presence at the briefings and sought to convince the president with the disingenuous argument that the peak of the pandemic had passed and, thus, there was no longer any reason for his daily presence at the briefings. These advisers were aided by the mention of disinfectant, it seems.

At a late April briefing, President Trump suggested that researchers should investigate whether injecting people with disinfectant could be an effective way to treat the coronavirus. The president rambled on about how it would knock out the virus in a minute. He ended his remarks by asking White House Coronavirus Task Force Coordinator Dr. Deborah Birx whether she had looked into injecting people with disinfectant. The look on Dr. Birx's face was, to say the least, interesting. The media and public uproar over seeming to suggest that we should inject people with disinfectant to treat the coronavirus may have rearranged the president's thinking about continuing the briefings. Surely the president's aides knew that when the president had gotten to the point of talking about injecting people with disinfectant, the daily briefings had jumped the shark.

But there was something else at work as well. As April soon became May, the president was becoming desperate to show that the crisis was ending and that everything was returning to normal. When he decided to end his daily briefings, the president's message focused on his personal grievances rather than any bold proclamation to the nation. A presidential tweet on April 25 explained his reasoning: "What is the purpose of having White House News Conferences when the Lamestream Media asks nothing but hostile questions, & then refuses to report the truth or facts accurately. They get record ratings, & the American people get nothing but Fake News. Not worth the time & effort!"

In the meantime, as the president was feeling somewhat sorry for himself, poison control centers were receiving a spike in phone calls following President Trump's suggestion that injecting people with disinfectant might help people infected with coronavirus. Soon the makers of Lysol were so alarmed that they felt compelled to issue a statement that emphasized "under no circumstance should our disinfectant products be administered into the human body (through injection, ingestion or any other route)."[50]

The *New York Times* published a report analyzing every word Donald Trump had spoken about the COVID-19 outbreak at the daily task force briefings that he now saw as "not worth the time & effort." Between March 9 and April 27, he had congratulated himself on his response to the coronavirus pandemic on almost every occasion. His statements and remarks were categorized into words of self-congratulations, exaggerations and falsehoods, crediting others, blaming others, and displaying empathy. Statements of self-congratulations were the most frequent. President Trump congratulated himself over 600 times. He credited others for their work some 360 times, and he blamed others 110 times. The president had tried, with very mixed success, to display empathy or appeal to national unity about 160 times.[51]

The level of self-congratulations that occurred every day at these press briefings was, in a word, stunning. They were the defining characteristic of the administration's response to a public health emergency. In no small measure, they did indeed make the briefings not worth the effort for an anxious public in need of scientifically sound information and wise direction. It was becoming abundantly clear that managing perceptions or appearances was the president's primary concern. Managing the pandemic response was never his first priority.

Conclusion

By June 1, long after most states had already begun to relax defensive restrictions, there had been 1,809,109 cases of coronavirus in the United States and at least 105,099 deaths in a little over three months.[52] Many Americans were having positive thoughts and high hopes about the "reopening" of the country. But if they reflected on what the first five months of 2020 had shown them and had been listening to any of what the experts had tried to communicate over the discordant rhythms of politics, the confusing and disjointed responses of fifty states, and the mixed messaging of one very inconsistent federal government, they would have had ample reason to fear what the coming months might yet bring. The first wave was not really over, as we would discover much to our chagrin, and the first five months were not the worst of it. The worst was not behind us. As we may remember hearing in February or March, if we were fortunate to be able to hear anyone who actually knew what they were talking about, this was a marathon and not a sprint.

The first five months of 2020 were frightening on several levels. A global pandemic was on the loose, and there was much Americans would learn about COVID-19 that would cause growing concern with the passage of each day. What they needed most as the pandemic became a reality in their daily lives was clear, accurate, and timely information based on the science delivered by trusted leaders in a manner that would inform and motivate people to make the best choices for themselves, their loved ones, and their communities. What they got instead could not but help to elevate their level of concern and fear.

Leaders at the national and state levels created conflicting narratives. Some were serious in following the science and implementing necessary defensive measures to slow the spread of the virus. Some, and especially the president of the United States, ignored, misrepresented, or simply confused the facts and ignored the science. The experts were, for the most part, reliable, and they provided wise counsel. But when leaders send messages contrary to those of the experts, it undermines them and strips fact-based evidence of its ability to influence public opinion and behavior. This leaves the public befuddled and not knowing whom to believe or what actions to take.

The confusion that typified the U.S. response to COVID-19 began with the lack of a coherent and science-based national strategy for responding to a pandemic. The discontinuation of the planning efforts that had advanced under the previous two administrations, including the shutting down of the NSC planning group and the weakening of public health agencies over the first three years of the Trump presidency, surely weakened U.S. preparedness for a major public health emergency. Still, the United States did have two months to anticipate and upgrade its preparedness for what was obviously headed its way. The Trump administration chose instead to rely on a containment strategy (i.e., travel restrictions) to keep COVID-19 out of the country. While such a step was arguably a step worth taking, it was not an answer to the challenge. What it might have done was buy time to prepare for the inevitable onslaught of the approaching storm. This would have meant ramping up the production and distribution of medical supplies and PPE in the national stockpile, working with the states to lay out an integrated and comprehensive plan of action, and preparing the American public for the steps that would have to be taken by every state in the nation as a part of truly national strategy. Instead, the administration perpetuated the false belief that the travel restrictions would do the job, painted a rosy picture ("everything is under control"), and provided no guidance to state and local governments.

As the virus began its spread across the nation, each state was left to decide for itself how to respond. This led to a hodgepodge of state actions and a disjointed effort that was inconsistent from one state to the next. Some states acted intelligently, some followed the lead of President Trump in downplaying the need to do anything, and all of them acted too late. The federal government was ineffective at providing any substantive and timely assistance to the states as they became swamped with cases. They were left to compete with each other for the PPE and other supplies they needed, and they were generally left to fend for themselves in the beginning.

Ideally, in a well-developed and properly implemented national strategy, the states would have been integrated into a national response. Rather than fifty states reacting to events and implementing response actions in a shotgun approach, they could have been organized to implement the same game plan. They could have, perhaps, been better enabled to anticipate what was coming and recognize the specific steps that needed to be taken. These steps could have been taken in a more coordinated manner that did not see their responses contradicting each other. A pandemic does not take note of state borders. If the virus is in one state, it will soon be in all states. The stay-at-home orders that most states ultimately implemented were an inevitability from the outset. That should have been made clear in any national strategy, and no governor should have felt that he or she was going to be able to avoid implementing one. More to the point, there needed to be better coordination between the states in implementing these orders to enhance the chances of flattening the curve or slowing the spread.

In fact, the best course would have been a complete national shutdown—a nationwide stay-at-home order. This would have needed to have been issued very early (perhaps early March), and it would have had to remain in effect for a full three months to have done the most good. Doing this on a state-by-state basis, and after the pandemic was already raging within a state's borders, was not nearly as effective a strategy. All of this would have required strong national leadership. At precisely the time such leadership would have done the most good, our president offered the wishful thinking that the virus would somehow miraculously disappear ("It will go away"). One of the scariest things about the first five months of 2020 was the apparent failure of the president as well as a number of state governors to grasp the science of a novel pathogen that was killing more Americans in less time than a major war might have done.

By the beginning of May, it did appear that many states had made progress in slowing the spread. The corner had not exactly been turned; there were still hot spots, and the nation's numbers with respect to both cases and deaths were still increasing. By May 3, over sixty-five thousand Americans had died of COVID-19. A Columbia University study reported that if the United States had adopted social distancing measures on March 8, nearly thirty-six thousand of those deaths could have been avoided. If the measures had begun on March 1, the study estimated almost fifty-four thousand deaths could have been spared.[53] As states began to reopen their economies and lift lockdowns, the scientists who authored the study said their findings underlined the need for a swift response when outbreaks begin to flare up. One would have to suspect that as the states reopened, there would be new flareups. Other studies also suggested that earlier action could have saved many thousands of lives. We will never really know for sure just how many lives might have been saved, but there can be no doubt that had we engaged aggressive mitigation measures earlier lives *would* have been saved.

In early May, states began the process of reopening after a couple of months on lockdown. Most Americans had supported the stay-at-home orders. Those who did not were often very vocal in expressing their displeasure. Even as states reopened, it was clear that there would be a need for some basic restrictions to be in place to prevent an unmanageable resurgence of infection. Many citizens would welcome such precautions, and others would chafe at them. Leadership would be required to guide the country through the narrow pathways that preserve individual liberty and yet serve to promote good health for all.

As states reopened their economies, there was undoubtedly a tendency in some quarters to believe that the pandemic was under control and that the first wave had ended. People could go back to work, businesses could reopen, and something approaching normal would return. Such supposition would, of course, entirely miss the point. We would still be living with coronavirus. We would still be living through a pandemic. We would most certainly be dealing with COVID-19 for some time. Were we prepared for that? Were our leaders prepared for that any more than they had been for the first wave? Was the first wave actually over? The next three months would provide the answers to these questions.

CHAPTER FIVE

The Great Reopening: Fools Rush In

There are more important things than living. And that's saving this country for my children and my grandchildren and saving this country for all of us.
—Texas Lt. Gov. Dan Patrick

Right now, we are preventing the spread of the disease by extreme social distancing, by keeping people away from each other. If we want to end that and let people interact with each other, we need to make sure infected people are not interacting with uninfected people. And the only way to know who is sick and pull them away from the uninfected is testing. That is literally Disease Outbreak 101.
—Dr. Ashish Jha, director of the Global Health Institute at Harvard University

Introduction

As states began the easing of stay-at-home lockdowns, many leading scientists expressed some understandable concerns. They worried that too many people in the reopening states and communities would interpret government guidelines at their own discretion. They worried that social distancing in too many reopened public gathering spots would be measured in centimeters. In bars and other gathering spots, it was a certainty that the shouting, guffawing, and face-to-face encounters would be a terrific time for COVID-19 to "party." Its transmission rate was sure to be very healthy in such environments. In short, there was more than a little concern that reopening would result in sheer madness. These concerns suggested that reopening our communities would need to be done carefully and based on metrics that science might tell us provide the greatest chance for success and a lower chance of sheer madness breaking out. This would also require leaders, at the national, state, and local levels, to be guided by science ahead of economics.

There is not a one-size-fits-all policy when it comes to reopening the economy in the middle of a pandemic. But there are some important metrics that would have to be used, to one extent or another, by policy makers at all levels for gradually ending lockdowns. There were three important metrics that would be emphasized by the experts. The first of these was hospital capacity. It must be remembered that one of the main purposes of the state stay-at-home orders was explicitly to flatten the curve so as not to overwhelm the local hospitals. This was essential so as not to deplete resources, including the human resources, needed to treat the ill. For any reopening of the economy to succeed, it was necessary to try to expand and maintain the capacity of local hospitals to be able to properly treat anyone who needed care. It was also necessary to minimize fatality rates.[1]

Assuming hospital capacity is adequate, geography-based metrics would be required. The COVID-19 virus spreads through human interaction. Relaxing stay-at-home orders and reopening communities meant interacting with people who may be infected. It was therefore important to know the number of infected people in the population. This meant massive testing, tracing, and targeted isolation. Testing was an especially important concern. To achieve its goal of providing accurate and timely information regarding the spread of the disease, it would be necessary to test everyone in a given community or region regularly (e.g., every couple of weeks). It was also important to make sure that those who tested positive entered and remained in isolation until they were confirmed as negative in a subsequent test. As the efforts to reopen the economy were beginning, there was more than ample reason to fear that the supply of diagnostic testing remained quite limited everywhere. According to Nobel Prize–winner Paul Romer, rolling out massive testing in the United States would require resources amounting to $100 billion. As of late June, well into the great American reopening, Congress had provided only $25 billion for testing. Much more would be needed.[2]

Tracking was another metric that the experts were saying was essential. This meant tracking the R0 (R-naught), or the average number of other people that an infected person would infect. If the R0 were to exceed one, this would mean that the disease was still spreading too rapidly. A number below one, which was the goal, would mean that the disease is contained and will eventually disappear. Tracking the daily R0 would have to be done on a state-by-state basis.[3] When the R0 of a state or a community is below one and is in a downward trend, the relaxing of social distancing measures would be in order. If the R0 were to rise again, state and local authorities would have a good measure to rely on to reimplement some lockdown policies as appropriate.

These three metrics of treatment (i.e., hospital capacity), testing, and tracing would be incorporated into most state and local reopening plans. The broadly accepted notion was that the reopening of the American economy needed to be phased, gradual, and safe. It was also important not to reopen too early or without strict attention paid to the data relevant to the "three T's" (testing, tracing, and treatment). It was understood that reopening would most likely spread the infection, especially if it were done recklessly or too quickly. Despite this general awareness, the fifty states implemented reopening plans that varied greatly. Some of this variance would be due to the differing conditions of each state with respect to each of the three metrics. Some of the variance, a good deal of it actually, would be due to the political inclinations of state and local officials and the degree of recklessness that this might entail. Once again, as in the response to the first wave and the issuance of stay-at-home orders, fifty different states marching to the beat of their own drummer, some in agreement with science and some in defiance of it, combined with the inadequacy of federal guidance and the lack of a national strategy to create confusion and inconsistency in the great reopening of America.

The Metrics and the Implementation: Reopening Nightmares

By the time most states had shut down in April, President Trump was already impatient to reopen the economy. As the nation was still in the acceleration phase of the pandemic, the president was not about to let the virus determine when the economy could safely reopen. That is what the experts were saying should happen, but for the president, the cure (shutdowns and stay-at-home orders) was worse than the disease. Initially, he said he wanted the economy to be reopened by Easter (late April). In the first week of May, with the first wave not nearly contained, his impatience to "reopen" the economy was a daily theme: "I'm not saying anything is perfect. And yes, will some people be affected? Yes. Will some people be affected badly? Yes. But we have to get our country open, and we have to get it open soon." Despite the fact that some people would be "affected badly," the president emphasized the need to get back to work to restore the U.S. economy, even if it meant some people might become sick or even die. As he was saying things like this, he visited a plant making protective face masks but did not wear one himself.[4] Critics suggested that Trump was so intent on having a good economy by Election Day that he prioritized reopening the economy ahead of doing what was necessary to contain the virus. Trump repeatedly insisted that the nation must return to business as usual within a timeline that was grossly unrealistic, at least insofar as infectious disease experts were concerned. It seemed as though he was ready to put the pandemic in his rearview mirror and simply avoid the public health problem that needed to be solved.

As the president and his economic advisers celebrated the fact that by the end of May almost every state had "reopened" its economy, an internal "situation update" from the Centers for Disease Control and Prevention (CDC) demonstrated some very serious concerns. The update included a chart projecting that the number of daily deaths caused by COVID-19 would steadily rise over the next month and reach about three thousand per day by June 1. This was roughly 70 percent more than the then current level (early May). When this internal report was leaked to the press, the White House was quick to distance itself from it. The president rejected the new projections, saying they had not even been submitted to or reviewed by the Coronavirus Task Force.[5] The administration wanted to pivot its messaging from fighting the virus to promoting the economy. With the end of the president's daily White House Coronavirus Task Force briefings at the end of April, the White House had shifted gears to boosting the economy and highlighting "success stories" of businesses while reducing its public emphasis or its reporting on health statistics.

Many experts expressed concern that the push to reopen the economy too quickly might ignite a resurgence of COVID-19 cases, sending the economy back into lockdown. They cautioned that the economy could not possibly "recover" until the pandemic was under control and advised that widespread reopening should wait for a sustained drop in death rates and a desperately needed enhancement in the availability of tests. They also stated that no one would be completely safe until a vaccine could be produced and widely distributed. That was still many months away.

As one might suspect during a public health crisis, the CDC developed some scientifically driven guidelines for states and communities as they began to reopen in the midst of a pandemic. During the first week of May, the CDC was ready to release an extensive report and a set of guidelines to provide local officials with step-by-step instructions for reopening public spaces during the coronavirus pandemic. This detailed document,

"Guidance for Implementing the Opening Up America Again Framework," would never see the light of day as far as the president was concerned. The White House shelved this report before it could be shared with the public. The president felt that these CDC guidelines were too restrictive and that they would slow the economic recovery from the impact of the state-by-state shutdowns that had been implemented.[6] The guidelines contained detailed advice for making site-specific decisions related to reopening businesses, schools, restaurants, summer camps, churches, day care centers, and other institutions. It also included detailed "decision trees" that would have been helpful to state and local governments and that would have helped to promote consistency in state-by-state efforts.[7]

The White House did allow the CDC to issue general and watered-down guidelines for the reopening of states. While not as detailed as the originally proposed guidelines, they were nevertheless helpful, or would have been helpful if properly and strictly implemented. It was entirely left up to state and local governments to voluntarily comply with the guidelines and to determine how to proceed. The proposed state and regional gating criteria, which suggested guidelines to be met before proceeding to a phased reopening, were sound, but they were not absolute. In other words, as the guidelines stated, "State and local officials may need to tailor the application of these criteria to local circumstances (e.g., metropolitan areas that have suffered severe COVID outbreaks, rural and suburban areas where outbreaks have not occurred or have been mild)."[8] This seemed to make the gating criteria more of a suggestion than a requirement. Nevertheless, it is worth taking a look at this criteria.

The first recommended criterion to be met before reopening was a downward trajectory of influenza-like illnesses reported within a fourteen-day period as well as a downward trajectory of COVID-like symptoms reported within a fourteen-day period. The second criterion was a downward trajectory of documented cases within a fourteen-day period. Failing that, there should at least be a downward trajectory of positive tests as a percent of total tests within a fourteen-day period (flat or increasing volume of tests). The third criterion was that hospitals should be able to treat all patients without crisis care, and there should be a robust testing program in place for at-risk health care workers, including emerging antibody testing.[9]

The less restrictive CDC guidelines that were released by the White House also recommended a phased approach to reopening. To begin the first phase of the reopening, states and regions were supposed to meet the "gating criteria." To proceed to the second stage, there should be no evidence of a spike in cases, and the gating criteria should be met a second time. To proceed to phase three, again, there should be no spike in cases, and states and regions would have to meet the gating criteria a third time. See box 5.1 for the specifics of each phase.

These White House–approved guidelines were less prescriptive than those originally proposed by the CDC. That may or may not have mattered, as many states forged ahead using their own standards. The result was predictably a patchwork of approaches, some stricter than the federal recommendations and many far less strict. For some states, it was easy to find real-time data on whether criteria had been satisfied. Other states seemed to go out of their way to make it more difficult to see where they stand on meeting their own criteria. Nevertheless, analysts concluded that *most states did not actually meet the gating criteria* before reopening.[10]

Box 5.1 Opening Up America: Three-Phased Approach

Phase One

For States and Regions that satisfy the gating criteria
INDIVIDUALS
ALL VULNERABLE INDIVIDUALS should continue to shelter in place. Members of households with vulnerable residents should be aware that by returning to work or other environments where distancing is not practical, they could carry the virus back home. Precautions should be taken to isolate from vulnerable residents.

All individuals, WHEN IN PUBLIC (e.g., parks, outdoor recreation areas, shopping areas), should maximize physical distance from others. Social settings of more than 10 people, where appropriate distancing may not be practical, should be avoided unless precautionary measures are observed.

Avoid SOCIALIZING in groups of more than 10 people in circumstances that do not readily allow for appropriate physical distancing (e.g., receptions, trade shows).

MINIMIZE NON-ESSENTIAL TRAVEL and adhere to CDC guidelines regarding isolation following travel.
EMPLOYERS
Continue to ENCOURAGE TELEWORK, whenever possible and feasible with business operations.

If possible, RETURN TO WORK IN PHASES.

Close COMMON AREAS where personnel are likely to congregate and interact or enforce strict social distancing protocols.

Minimize NON-ESSENTIAL TRAVEL and adhere to CDC guidelines regarding isolation following travel.

Strongly consider SPECIAL ACCOMMODATIONS for personnel who are members of a VULNERABLE POPULATION.

SPECIFIC TYPES OF EMPLOYERS

SCHOOLS AND ORGANIZED YOUTH ACTIVITIES (e.g., daycare, camp) that are currently closed should remain closed.

VISITS TO SENIOR LIVING FACILITIES AND HOSPITALS should be prohibited. Those who do interact with residents and patients must adhere to strict protocols regarding hygiene.

LARGE VENUES (e.g., sit-down dining, movie theaters, sporting venues, places of worship) can operate under strict physical distancing protocols.

ELECTIVE SURGERIES can resume, as clinically appropriate, on an outpatient basis at facilities that adhere to CMS guidelines.

GYMS can open if they adhere to strict physical distancing and sanitation protocols.

BARS should remain closed.

Phase Two

For States and Regions with no evidence of a rebound and that satisfy the gating criteria a second time

INDIVIDUALS

ALL VULNERABLE INDIVIDUALS should continue to shelter in place. Members of households with vulnerable residents should be aware that by returning to work or other environments where distancing is not practical, they could carry the virus back home. Precautions should be taken to isolate from vulnerable residents.

All individuals, WHEN IN PUBLIC (e.g., parks, outdoor recreation areas, shopping areas), should maximize physical distance from others. Social settings of more than 50 people, where appropriate distancing may not be practical, should be avoided unless precautionary measures are observed.

NON-ESSENTIAL TRAVEL can resume.

EMPLOYERS

Continue to ENCOURAGE TELEWORK, whenever possible and feasible with business operations.

Close COMMON AREAS where personnel are likely to congregate and interact, or enforce moderate social distancing protocols.

Strongly consider SPECIAL ACCOMMODATIONS for personnel who are members of a VULNERABLE POPULATION.

SPECIFIC TYPES OF EMPLOYERS

SCHOOLS AND ORGANIZED YOUTH ACTIVITIES (e.g., daycare, camp) can reopen.

VISITS TO SENIOR CARE FACILITIES AND HOSPITALS should be prohibited. Those who do interact with residents and patients must adhere to strict protocols regarding hygiene.

LARGE VENUES (e.g., sit-down dining, movie theaters, sporting venues, places of worship) can operate under moderate physical distancing protocols.

ELECTIVE SURGERIES can resume, as clinically appropriate, on an outpatient and in-patient basis at facilities that adhere to CMS guidelines.

GYMS can remain open if they adhere to strict physical distancing and sanitation protocols.

BARS may operate with diminished standing-room occupancy, where applicable and appropriate.

Phase Three

For States and Regions with no evidence of a rebound and that satisfy the gating criteria a third time

INDIVIDUALS

VULNERABLE INDIVIDUALS can resume public interactions, but should practice physical distancing, minimizing exposure to social settings where distancing may not be practical, unless precautionary measures are observed.

LOW-RISK POPULATIONS should consider minimizing time spent in crowded environments.

EMPLOYERS

Resume UNRESTRICTED STAFFING of worksites.

SPECIFIC TYPES OF EMPLOYERS

VISITS TO SENIOR CARE FACILITIES AND HOSPITALS can resume. Those who interact with residents and patients must be diligent regarding hygiene.

LARGE VENUES (e.g., sit-down dining, movie theaters, sporting venues, places of worship) can operate under limited physical distancing protocols.

GYMS can remain open if they adhere to standard sanitation protocols.

BARS may operate with increased standing-room occupancy.

Source: White House, https://www.whitehouse.gov/openingamerica/

As the great reopening began in states across the country in May, many plunged ahead without meeting the "suggested" benchmarks. Soon the Federal Emergency Management Agency (FEMA) began to adjust forecasts for the coronavirus death toll. By June 1, it was expected that American deaths would top three thousand per day. The national lockdown (i.e., stay-at-home orders) had been meant to reduce the spread of disease. An inevitable side effect of the lockdown was almost forty million Americans out of work, thousands of small businesses boarded up, and the worst economic crisis since the Great Depression of the previous century.

A heated national debate had erupted by the beginning of May. The two tragedies (i.e., the pandemic and the economic crisis) were seemingly pitted against each other. Instead of seeing the two as connected and realizing that the solution to the economic crisis required first resolving the public health crisis, the ensuing debate only left us with tragic choices. Americans seriously debated how many lives they were willing to spend in exchange for jobs, their livelihoods, and their ability to pay their bills. Lieutenant Governor Dan Patrick of Texas may not have spoken for most, but many did agree with his suggestion that old people should be willing to die to save the economy. "What I said when I was with you that night is there are more important things than living. And that's saving this country for my children and my grandchildren and saving this country for all of us," Patrick said. "I don't want to die, nobody wants to die, but man we've got to take some risks and get back in the game and get this country back up and running."[11]

President Trump was among those pushing the hardest to reopen the economy as quickly as possible. This was not a data-driven, scientifically justified priority; it was a political priority for him. He was desperate, given a decline in his polls, to juice the economy before the November election. As the push to reopen was spreading, and as fifty states seemed to be moving in fifty different directions with little federal guidance, Dr. Anthony Fauci testified before a Senate committee. As a leading member of the president's Coronavirus Task Force, he recommended caution. Reopening things too quickly (i.e., relaxing social-distancing restrictions too abruptly) would result in "multiple outbreaks throughout the country," Fauci said. He emphasized that this would "result in needless suffering and death."[12] Dr. Fauci is, of course, an infectious disease expert. But the president and many Republican governors were often not all that interested in what the experts had to say. Experts at leading universities, the American Enterprise Institute, and within the federal government had laid out detailed steps that would have helped the United States track

the spread of the disease in our communities, clamp down on new outbreaks, and arrive at data-driven decisions to facilitate a safe reopening.
The president and the fifty states followed their recommendations hap-
hazardly at best.

As states began to reopen, public health officials insisted that the only
way to contain future outbreaks was through dogged disease surveillance.
This meant that officials must identify not only people who have been
infected but also those with whom they have come into contact. Yet, the
United States had failed to develop a comprehensive contact tracing program as the great reopening began. The federal government had also left
the states pretty much on their own when it came to testing. State governments, in partnership with universities, researchers, and the National
Guard, tried to take up the slack. This would not overcome the disarray
and slowness of the federal government to ramp up support for expanded
testing. When it came to testing, American efforts were embarrassingly
meager when compared with those of other advanced nations.[13] In May, as
the states began to reopen, the United States should have been conducting
forty million to fifty million tests every month to provide the basic minimal surveillance on the spread of the disease in this country, but it would
take until at least September to reach those numbers. The United States
was months behind where it needed to be for a safe reopening.[14]

Any prospects for a successful and safe reopening of the United States
were irreparably damaged by President Trump himself. After all, the president had repeatedly undermined the guidance of his own public health
officials, supported and even promoted anti-quarantine protests on his
Twitter account, and politicized the more data-based and cautious positions taken by some Democratic governors. Now, as the reopening was
underway, the president and his administration buried more detailed
CDC advice on how to safely reopen. His political response to the public
health crisis meant that he and his many supporters, including some governors, would disregard the science and refuse to embrace an incremen-
tal, data-driven approach to reopening. Public health experts were saying
that the United States would have a better outcome if the reopening was
implemented more gradually and much more carefully. The successes of
other countries in following that more gradual and careful approach demonstrated that it would work.[15] What would unfold over the next three
months was an inevitable train wreck.

The states to reopen the quickest, and most recklessly if the truth be
told, were typically the states that had closed the latest and where Republican governors had downplayed the pandemic and emphasized their
concerns about the economy. By the end of July, many of these states,

particularly in the Sunbelt, found themselves reversing course as their cases surged and their hospitals filled up past the breaking point. Beaches and bars that had reopened and were jam-packed for Memorial Day had to shut back down for the Fourth of July. Face masks, despite the earlier reluctance of many conservative state and local leaders to embrace the wearing of them, would soon be required in many states and on all airlines. Governors in several states that were among the hardest hit in the opening months of the pandemic, and whose states had reopened more cautiously and with better results, soon required travelers from the new hot zones to self-quarantine upon arrival. School districts and universities began reevaluating plans for opening in the fall, thus kicking off another heated debate about priorities.

If we consider that it was the end of April when the process of reopening began to unfold, the raw case and death toll numbers (see table 5.1) over the next three months tell an interesting story. First, Dr. Fauci was correct to be worried about "multiple outbreaks throughout the country" that might "result in needless suffering and death" if the reopening was not done in a cautious and safe manner.[16] Second, the "first wave" never really ended. It can be suggested that the rush to reopen and the manner in which the reopening occurred perpetuated and accelerated the first wave in the United States.

From the time that states began the rush to reopen, in late April, both case numbers and the death toll would continue to soar. In roughly the first month of reopening, the cases doubled from one million to two million. The death toll also doubled from 50,000 to 100,000. The next two months (June and July) saw the case rate double again (from two million to four million), and the death toll mounted from 100,000 on May 27 to 148,915 on July 26. Led by a spike in outbreaks in the South and West, the second peak of confirmed cases in the pandemic's first U.S. wave surpassed what was thought to be the initial peak in April. Most of the states that had jumped out early in April to start the great reopening were forced to pause or begin to roll back their reopening by July.

Georgia's stay-at-home order had expired on April 30, but Republican Governor Brian Kemp began reopening the state days before. Restaurants, personal care businesses, gyms, theaters, bowling alleys, and private social clubs were all allowed to reopen under some minimal restrictions. At this same time, North Carolina's Democratic Governor Roy Cooper and President Trump were at war over planning for the Republican National Convention scheduled to be held in that state. The Republican Party had a contract with North Carolina to host its national convention in Charlotte in late August, but President Trump said he might look for

Table 5.1   U.S. COVID-19 Cases and Deaths: April 28–July 26, 2020

Cumulative Cases by Date	
April 28	1 million cases
June 1	2 million cases
July 1	3 million cases
July 23	4 million cases
American COVID-19 Death Toll	
April 28	50,000
May 27	100,000
July 26	148,915

Source: Johns Hopkins University, *USA Today*, https://www.usatoday.com/story/news
/nation/2020/07/23/united-states-coronavirus-cases-deaths-timeline/5485674002/

another venue if Governor Cooper did not guarantee the event could be held at full capacity. The governor insisted that his decision would be driven by the number of coronavirus cases and that, in all probability, attendance would have to be very limited.

As the president and the Republican Party searched for an alternative venue, Georgia's Governor Kemp was quick to promote his state as an alternative site. There had been suggestions that Georgia had massaged virus data to justify an early reopening. It seemed that Georgia officials had been presenting data in a way that made the state appear healthier than it was. They had been one of the last states to shut down and, after only three weeks, were the first to reopen. By mid-July, the state's seven-day rolling average of newly reported cases was 3,507. This was quadruple its April pre-shutdown peak.[17]

As the summer surge of cases mounted in Georgia, the City of Atlanta and other cities issued face mask requirements, but the governor would have none of it. He issued an order voiding all coronavirus mask orders issued by local governments around the state, but the City of Atlanta refused to comply. The governor then took the extreme step of filing a lawsuit to block the City of Atlanta's mask requirement. In addition to doubting that masks provided any protection against spread of the coronavirus, Governor Kemp emphasized that "mask mandates are unenforceable." While saying that he trusted Georgians to wear masks without an ordinance, he added that "what people should be thinking about are the livelihoods of the businesses. We're already in a very tough position, we have got to balance both of those things. We cannot be afraid of this virus."[18]

In Florida, Republican Governor Ron DeSantis had relented and issued a stay-at-home order on April 3. But by May 4, he too was willing and eager to move quickly to reopen the state. As early as April 17, some municipalities were allowed to reopen parks and beaches with social distancing guidelines in place. As the next few weeks proceeded, Florida reopened the rest of the state very quickly. This brought about expert predictions that there would be a serious uptick in COVID cases throughout the state. Governor DeSantis insisted that such predictions were the work of political critics who wanted to raise the alarm and that they were wrong. The governor was so confident that the virus would just go away that he succeeded in luring the Republican National Convention from North Carolina to Florida. He promised a "full house," without restrictions, in Jacksonville. In a phone conversation with President Trump, DeSantis said he would not require masks and that the virus would not be a major problem in August in Florida.[19]

But the virus soon spread out of control in Florida. This was largely due, of course, to decision-making shaped by politics and divorced from scientific expertise. By the end of July, Florida was near the breaking point. By that time, fifty-eight hundred Floridians had died of COVID-19, and one out of every fifty-two Floridians had been infected with the virus. The state's hospitals and intensive care units were being pushed to the brink, Florida's unemployment system was overwhelmed, and its tourism industry was in complete shambles. By the end of July, Florida had topped New York's April numbers and stood as the epicenter of the pandemic. In mid-July, all planning for a splashy and jam-packed Republican National Convention in Jacksonville was halted. The convention was subsequently canceled.[20]

Texas was another all-too-familiar story. In March, as cases of the new coronavirus began to pop up in Texas cities, Republican Governor Greg Abbott remained fairly passive. He deferred to local officials and resisted calls for a statewide stay-at-home order. He expressed his view that "local officials have the authority to implement more strict standards. . . . I would applaud them for doing so."[21] As cases mounted, Abbott finally did take statewide action. He issued an order for Texans to remain in place except for essential activities, such as grocery shopping. The goal was to slow the spread of the virus. Cases rose steadily throughout the month of April, but things did seem to be improving just a bit. Texas was adding fewer than one thousand new cases per day.

Many of Governor Abbott's fellow Texan Republicans grew restless very quickly. Lieutenant Governor Dan Patrick was making national headlines for telling Fox News, "There are more important things than living." The president had said he wanted the economy "opened up and raring to go" by Easter. As a result, just as Abbott had reluctantly shut the state down, he immediately began to talk about reopening. He announced that businesses would reopen in phases starting May 1. This reopening would be phased in stages, but unlike in some states, there were few specific health metrics that controlled the reopening process. To the experts, this meant that the pandemic could well spiral out of control in Texas, and events soon warranted that concern. On April 30, the day before the reopening commenced, Texas reported its highest death toll up to that time.[22] As the bars and restaurants were reopened, the case numbers soared.

When the CDC began recommending the wearing of masks in April, Abbott also encouraged Texans to wear masks. But this would remain a recommendation only. There would be no state order regarding face masks. He also stripped local leaders, such as mayors and county judges, of the ability to mandate stronger restrictions, including the wearing of masks. By June, Abbott had acknowledged that the virus was spreading at an "unacceptable rate." Days later, he paused the state's reopening process, closed the bars again, and told Texans, "There's never a reason for you to have to leave your home." Restaurants remained open, and the governor appeared before a gathering of hundreds at a Dallas church. Another featured guest, Vice President Mike Pence, also spoke at this gathering.

Predictably, Texas was soon overwhelmed with coronavirus cases. The familiar scenes of refrigerated trucks to hold the dead and overcrowded medical facilities became common. A surge of COVID-19 deaths in rural Texas forced one hospital to set up "death panels" to decide which patients could be saved and which ones would be sent home to die.[23] The governor was soon opining that he regretted that he may have opened up the state too early. In neighboring Arizona, a similar crisis was unfolding.

Arizona's Republican Governor Doug Ducey, who had issued a stay-at-home order in April, was also eager to reopen the state. He said that his decision to reopen was based on science, not politics. At the same time, as he reopened the state, state health officials told a team of university experts to stop working on models that projected what would happen next. These models had shown that the only way to avoid a dramatic spike in cases was to delay reopening the state until the end of May. Tim Lant, a mathematical epidemiologist at Arizona State University, warned, "It's not safe to reopen unless you're planning on, you know, shutting down again after a couple of weeks."[24] Lant and his team were subsequently informed that their services were no longer needed. They would also be cut off from access to state data they needed to continue their modeling.

As of June 20, Arizona had recorded 46,689 coronavirus cases. Ten days later, the state reported over 75,000 cases. These numbers would continue to get much worse. The largest increase was from those between the ages of twenty and forty-four, those whom one might have predicted would be the most socially active as the state quickly reopened. At the end of June, the governor implemented one of the most drastic rollbacks of reopening that any state had yet ordered. Bars, gyms, movie theaters, and other businesses were closed again for thirty days. Public events with more than fifty people were prohibited. Restaurants were allowed to remain open with physical distancing guidelines in place. Although recommending that citizens wear face masks, the governor would not issue a state requirement that they be worn. Governor Ducey also said he would not require people attending President Donald Trump's Phoenix rally on June 23 to wear masks.[25] By July 30, there were 170,798 confirmed cases of coronavirus and 3,626 coronavirus-related deaths reported in Arizona. Along with Florida, Georgia, and Texas, Arizona was a poster child for failed reopenings.

One must note that caseloads were not just exploding in Republican-led states. The state of California had been praised for its timely and successful efforts in March and April to slow the spread of the coronavirus outbreak, and it had been regarded as one of the success stories in the spring. However, by midsummer, it too was experiencing an explosion of new cases. Governor Gavin Newsom, a Democrat, had issued the nation's first statewide stay-at-home order, and he had earned praise for his timely action. Experts said that the stay-at-home order had been a big success. But the subsequent reopening of the state was not a big success.

In May, California officials began to rapidly reopen businesses. The people of California, like people all across the country, had been pent up in their homes and were eager to get back to routines. The economic damage inevitably caused by the state shutdowns also contributed to the urgency many felt about the need to reopen. Predictably, as California reopened, coronavirus hospitalizations in California began accelerating around June 15 at a rate not seen since early April. Public health officials noted that indoor dining and drinking posed a more significant public health risk than other retail activities, even with social distancing. Officials in Los Angeles County found that many establishments were not following safety protocols. At the end of June, it was reported that 49 percent of bars and 33 percent of restaurants were not adhering to physical distancing protocols indoors, and 54 percent of bars and 44 percent of restaurants were not enforcing mask and face shield requirements. Soon, local communities were forced to once again shutter gyms, houses of worship, malls, and businesses. By June, Governor Newsom had issued orders requiring all Californians to wear masks or other face coverings while in public or in high-risk settings. By early July, California had seen more than 333,000 confirmed cases and more than 7,000 coronavirus-related deaths. After its early success, it was clear that a rapid reopening had led to a second closing in a relatively short period of time.[26]

By the end of July, new coronavirus outbreaks had spread across much of the nation. These outbreaks did not discriminate between states that had proceeded wisely or recklessly to reopen. Regardless of how the states had proceeded, it was beginning to appear that reopenings had been too rushed in too many cases. On July 28, twenty-one states were said to be in the "red zone" for coronavirus outbreaks under federal criteria, meaning they had reported more than one hundred new cases per one hundred thousand people in the previous week. Those states were Alabama, Arizona, Arkansas, California, Florida, Georgia, Idaho, Iowa, Kansas, Louisiana, Mississippi, Missouri, Nevada, North Carolina, North Dakota, Oklahoma, South Carolina, Tennessee, Texas, Utah, and Wisconsin. The CDC said that this would call for further restrictions in the states listed. President Trump, true to his science-avoidance form, called for more states to continue reopening the day after the CDC's release. During a visit to North Carolina to promote vaccine research, the president said that "a lot of the governors should be opening up states that they're not opening, and we'll see what happens with them."[27]

Of course, the whole discussion of reopening, the debates about how fast to reopen, and the president's urging for a faster reopening were distractions from what the case and death toll numbers were actually telling us: the United States had failed to control the virus because its leaders and citizens had not followed the basics of outbreak response. As unimaginable as it may seem, the United States stood alone among advanced nations in its inability to manage the pandemic crisis. It simply seemed to be incapable of getting ahead of the virus and controlling its spread.

Mixed Messages, Mixed Behaviors, Cultural Wars, and Failure

Mixed messages and misinformation proved to be as highly contagious as COVID-19 itself. As the world engaged in a battle to contain the virus and to find a treatment and a vaccine for it, the United States was unique in its disorganized national leadership, its outbreak of coronavirus conspiracy theories, its anti-mask myths, and its sham cures. Combined with its ongoing partisan and cultural warfare, these things more or less preordained that the United States would fail to meet the challenge. There was simply no antidote for the outbreaks of coronavirus conspiracy theories. There was no preventative cure for the impact of misinformation and mixed messaging coming out of the mouth of the president and out of the mouths of many others in positions of national and state leadership. In addition to battling the coronavirus, experts also had to battle a torrent of misleading information that undermined their best efforts to slow the spread of the virus. The experts struggled to get the message to the public about what they could do to protect themselves. They sought to convey the best scientific guidance to protect public health. As they did so, more and more people put themselves in harm's way because they refused to believe that the virus was something they had to deal with or worry about.

Why did so many decide not to believe the experts? Fed by mixed messages from a variety of sources, it was hard for many to know what to believe. Messages contrary to the expert advice were transmitted by social media, amplified by the president and other leaders, mutating when confronted by contradictory facts, and ceaseless in their bombardment. Sadly, the "leadership" of President Trump would be one of the most important factors that enhanced the influence of misinformation.

There is a very great danger in providing politically motivated or inaccurate information to the public during a pandemic. Under such circumstances, people will either panic or disregard the public health crisis. They will lose confidence in their government or they will simply elect not to take any safeguards to protect themselves from something that seems to be a matter in dispute. A summary of the many times President Trump contradicted public health experts suggests that he was patient zero (i.e., the first to be infected with a disease) in what could only be called a "misinformation pandemic." Recalling the almost daily barrage of presidential misstatements in the daily newsfeeds, one could not help but be overwhelmed with evidence of the president's malady.

As the new coronavirus emerged and the CDC declared it to be a pandemic and U.S. public health experts warned of the dangers ahead, the president sought to politicize the pandemic. First, as he told his cheering supporters during a campaign rally, the pandemic was the next "Democrat hoax." He repeatedly asserted in public statements and tweets that the state stay-at-home orders were a political strategy by Democrats to slow down the economy and ruin his reelection chances. He said, even during the peak of the summer outbreaks, that the Democratic governors would reopen the states on November 4 (the day after the election). In other words, he persistently presented the message that the measures taken by state and local officials (especially Democrats) to stop the spread of the virus were part of some political strategy or conspiracy to harm him. Needless to say, many of his ardent followers were easily persuaded.

Beyond his campaign rallies and daily tweet storms, President Trump consistently contradicted, or was contradicted by, his own and a variety of other public health experts. In March, he claimed that testing for the new virus was "going very smooth" as he asserted that "anybody that needs a test can get one." The tests themselves were said to be "beautiful" or "perfect." He would be contradicted by Alex Azar, his secretary of Health and Human Services, who noted that you could not get a test unless a doctor prescribed one. Dr. Anthony Fauci was more direct in congressional testimony, saying that the United States was not where it needed to be with regard to testing. He noted that it was not as easy as it should be to get tested.

Early on, President Trump insisted that the new coronavirus was no more serious than the seasonal flu. He repeatedly claimed that the virus was being contained, even predicting in March that it would disappear one day "like a miracle." As public health officials were warning of millions of infections, the president said we would be nowhere close to that. "We're going very substantially down, not up," he said with regard to infections. "When you have 15 people and the 15 within a couple of days is going to be close to zero, that's a pretty good job we've done." Dr. Fauci provided a more sober assessment in later testimony to Congress as he warned that things were almost certainly going to get worse. President Trump insisted during a phone interview with Sean Hannity that the WHO's estimated death rate for coronavirus was a "false number." He said he had a "hunch" about this. A few days later, on March 9, the president tweeted that the coronavirus was no more lethal than the seasonal flu: "So last year 37,000 Americans died from the common flu. It averages between 27,000 and 70,000 per year, nothing is shut down, life & the economy go on. . . . Think about that!" These instances of the president seemingly downplaying the seriousness of the virus, contradicting experts, and politicizing the pandemic response did not end with the spring. Summer saw the virus spread without interruption, and all of the president's rosy assertions were proven to be 100 percent wrong.

As the American case numbers and death totals increased throughout the summer, it was clear that the United States had failed to contain the spread of the pandemic. It was alone among the advanced countries in this failure. On August 1, for example, the coronavirus death total for that single day (Spain 0, Germany 0, France 11, Australia 7, Japan 12, United

States 1,244) demonstrated just how exceptional the United States was in the context of this pandemic. Why was the United States so much less successful than European nations in containing the virus? Dr. Anthony Fauci, once again testifying before a congressional committee, explained that the drop in European cases was a result of those countries shutting down up to 95 percent of their economies; the United States only shut down 50 percent. The president disagreed and, inevitably, criticized Dr. Fauci. He claimed the reason U.S. cases continued to spike had to do with testing. The president asserted that if we tested less, there would be fewer cases. The president was, of course, 100 percent wrong. Dr Fauci was correct in asserting that the difference between shutdowns was the critical variable. He was also correct in observing that while some states followed the CDC guidelines in reopening, others did not. This contributed to the surges in many western and southern states. President Trump tweeted, among other things, that Dr. Fauci was a "fraud."

To the president's frequent distortion of facts and contradictions of what public health experts were saying, one must add the distortions and contradictions echoed by leading Republican figures in Congress and many state governors. Republican congressional members and state legislatures were refusing to wear masks, even though the CDC said that this was a necessary thing to control the spread of the virus. In some cases, they also suggested that the pandemic was a hoax or a political conspiracy by Democrats to weaken the president's reelection chances. In many cases, they were the leading voices in opposition to state stay-at-home orders and were quick to ignore CDC guidelines for the safe reopening of the economy. In some states, Republican state legislators sought to prevent Democratic governors from issuing stay-at-home orders, face mask requirements, and other restrictions to slow the spread. Given the political divisions that were on display as our "leaders" failed to present a united front in responding to the pandemic, it is no wonder that the American public was similarly divided. At the very least, they were understandably confused. They would also be all the more susceptible to the many baseless theories exploding on social media.

One baseless theory alleged that coronavirus was not real. Another claimed it was a bioweapon that had been created by adversaries of the United States or even by the U.S. government itself. In the early months of the outbreak, one was apt to come across the conspiracy theory that Microsoft founder Bill Gates was planning to use COVID-19 vaccines to implant microchips in all seven billion humans on the planet. Another claimed that doctors, journalists, and federal officials were joining forces to lie about the threat to hurt President Trump politically. The flood of such nonsense on social media only needed a few believers to make a chaotic response even more chaotic. To these crackpot theories may be added the common misperceptions that many people entertained even after the science and the experts proved otherwise.

Many young people assumed that they need not worry about the pandemic. It was, they thought, more of a threat to older people and not a deadly threat to them. This led to the scenes of young people crowding bars, beaches, and other social gatherings with reckless abandon as states reopened. The spikes in infections over the summer months were fueled by a rapidly expanding number of younger people testing positive. Many people seemed not to understand the basics of how the disease was actually transmitted. Public health experts would spend months emphasizing that face masks were the most effective tool we had to fight the pandemic, yet many people refused to wear them. The war over face masks is a prime example of misinformation combining with politics and the lack of effective national leadership to fan the flames of the pandemic.

The World Health Organization (WHO) updated its guidance about the wearing of face masks on June 5. It reported that the developing science had proven the effectiveness of face mask protection as a weapon against the virus. The WHO advised all nations to wear fabric face coverings wherever the coronavirus was spreading. The CDC reported that the science had conclusively shown that wearing face masks would protect both the wearer and others from COVID-19, and it urged everyone to wear a face mask when around other people in public. President Trump was reluctant to wear a face mask in public, even after he eventually (over four million U.S. cases and 150,000 U.S. deaths into the pandemic) came around to recommend that others do so. Early on, the president and many of his allies actually opined that people only wore masks to express their disapproval of the president. The wearing of a face mask, a public health measure, was inevitably and with tragic consequences made into something political. Despite that, by August 1, at least thirty-nine states had put some form of mask requirement in place. The spike in new cases left them no choice. President Trump opposed any national requirement regarding face masks, saying people should have a "certain freedom." Republican governors in Florida, Georgia, Arizona, and Texas also continued to oppose the issuing of any state face mask requirements.

By late summer, it was apparent that many Americans had not yet gotten the message that their breath could be lethal to another person. They had not yet accepted the fact that wearing a mask would make a very big difference in helping to stop the transmission of the disease. In part, they did not get this message because it was never properly and convincingly articulated by national and, in many cases, state leadership. The messaging was mixed and chaotic. It left too much room for debate when what was called for was an unequivocal and precise public health guideline. Some may have said, "The president doesn't wear a face mask, so why should I?" The president may have thought that his not wearing a mask was a sign of strength. However, it could more accurately be described as a failure of leadership. It was one of the many things that contributed to mixed behavior across the nation.

Many Americans entered grocery stores wearing a mask, but then they saw others refusing to do so. "Why do these people not see that they may be putting the rest of us in danger," they wondered. Someone not wearing a mask may have been thinking, "I'm young and healthy. So what if I get infected. I will be fine." Of course, even young and healthy people are a very important part in the chain of transmission to other people of all ages. It was another message not received. For some Americans, the thinking was that wearing a mask was a violation of their individual freedom. Not wearing a mask was, for them, a symbol of individualism. There were also those who refused to wear a mask because they thought wearing one was a sign of liberalism or socialism.

According to a June 2020 Pew Research Center survey, 65 percent of U.S. adults said that they had personally worn a mask or face covering in stores or other businesses all or most of the time (see table 5.2). A relatively small number of adults said they hardly ever (9 percent) or never (7 percent) wore a mask. But the survey did confirm that, to some extent, the wearing of face masks had become a partisan issue. Democrats and those who lean Democratic were more likely than Republicans and Republican-leaning respondents to say they personally wore a mask all or most of the time. Conservative Republicans were among the least likely to say they had worn a mask all or most of the time (49 percent).[28]

Despite the fact that 80 percent of all adults claimed to be wearing face coverings most or some of the time, those surveyed in the June 4–10 Pew study reported that mask-wearing behavior as they observed it in their communities was not quite that robust. About six in ten adults (62 percent) who lived in counties with the highest COVID-19 death rates said that all or most of the people in their communities were wearing masks, compared with 33 percent of those who lived in areas that had the lowest number of coronavirus deaths per capita. Those living in urban and suburban communities (63 percent and 68 percent, respectively) were much more likely than those living in rural areas (43 percent) to say they saw all or most people wearing masks.[29] It must also be noted that those who refused to wear masks or face coverings, despite being fewer in number,

Table 5.2   Wearing of Masks in Stores or Businesses

**Percent of People Who Say They Have Worn Masks or Face Coverings
Survey Conducted June 4–10, 2020**

	All/Most of Time	Some of the Time	Net
All adults	65%	15%	80%
Republican	53%	19%	72%
Democrat	76%	12%	88%
White	62%	16%	78%
Black	69%	17%	86%
Hispanic	74%	13%	87%
Asian	80%	9%	89%

Source: Pew Research Center, https://www.pewresearch.org/fact-tank/2020/06/23
/most-americans-say-they-regularly-wore-a-mask-in-stores-in-the-past-month-fewer-see
-others-doing-it/

were increasingly vocal and in some cases threatening. Many frontline
workers in various places of business reported violent reactions (i.e.,
being spit upon, threatened with violence, or verbally abused) from customers who refused to wear face masks where they were required.

By the beginning of August, as more and more states had issued face
mask requirements, two-thirds of Americans reported wearing a mask at
all times when leaving the home, even as other social distancing measures fell by the wayside. An Axios-Ipsos poll released in the first week of
August reported that 67 percent of Americans said they were wearing a
mask at all times. This included 48 percent of Republicans. Yet, only 21
percent reported wearing a mask at all times during their visits with
friends or family, potentially limiting the effectiveness of wearing a mask.
Interestingly, 35 percent reported that they had gone out to eat in the previous week. At about this time, one could also observe that there were a
growing number of sizable private gatherings where social distancing was
not observed and other safety protocols (i.e., mask wearing) were not
always observed.[30]

Other interesting findings in the Axios-Ipsos poll included the number
of Americans who had a "personal connection" to COVID-19 and the
declining level of trust citizens had in the federal government. Almost
half of Americans (46 percent) said they knew someone who had tested
positive for coronavirus, and half of that number (49 percent) knew
someone in their immediate community who had tested positive. Addi-
tionally, 17 percent of those surveyed reported that they had been tested.

More ominously, about one in five Americans said they knew someone who had died due to the coronavirus. About 4 percent of all Americans reported that the person who died was a family member, and 8 percent of Black and Hispanic respondents reported knowing a family member who had died. This personal experience of the disease was undoubtedly one of the factors that influenced the sagging confidence level of the American people with respect to the federal response. Only 29 percent of Americans said they had a fair amount or great deal of trust in the federal government to look out for the best interests of them and their families. By the first week of August, confidence in the federal government had reached a new low.[31]

At the beginning of August, new surveys showed that fewer than one-third of Americans said they trusted what President Donald Trump had said about the coronavirus, while a majority of the public trusted the messaging from the country's leading health experts. Actually, most Americans did not trust the president, and most Republicans did not trust the public health experts (see table 5.3). The pandemic was indeed a partisan issue. This is the last thing a pandemic should be, from a public health standpoint. Yet, one should not be surprised that it became a partisan matter. That is precisely a function of President Trump's "leadership." At the beginning of July, Dr. Fauci, whom you will remember had led the National Institute of Allergy and Infectious Diseases since the HIV/AIDS crisis in the 1980s, had warned that COVID-19 cases were beginning to climb in July and would continue to do so. White House officials responded, at the direction of their leader, by providing reporters with a list of times they claimed Dr. Fauci had made mistakes during the pandemic. The president himself retweeted a message calling for Fauci's firing, although he sought to tamp down concerns that this inevitably raised. When the president of the United States seeks to discredit his public health experts in the middle of a pandemic, it only serves to create conflict and widen the partisan divide at a time when national unity is required to address a national crisis. The pandemic was a partisan issue by presidential design.

The president's overall job approval rating had declined over the summer; only 31 percent of Americans trusted his handling of the pandemic. With an eye on the fast-approaching November presidential election, the president's staff (having changed their mind since the spring) persuaded him to resume the daily White House coronavirus briefings. The thinking was that he needed to be seen to be in charge and on top of all developments. In short, he needed to market himself as being in charge and boldly working the problem.

Table 5.3   Who Do Americans Trust on COVID-19?

	All	Republicans	Independents	Democrats
Percent trusting president	31%	69%	13%	2%
Percent trusting Dr. Fauci	51%	32%	40%	78%
Percent trusting the CDC	55%	38%	49%	76%
Percent trusting their state governor	49%	41%	40%	63%

Source: NBC News|SurveyMonkey Weekly Tracking Poll, August 4, 2020, https://www
.nbcnews.com/politics/2020-election/poll-americans-don-t-trust-trump-coronavirus
-republicans-don-t-n1235680

In all honesty, the president had disengaged from any interest in the managing of the pandemic. His focus had been, since the end of the briefings in the spring, on reopening the economy and returning to normalcy. The pandemic would "just go away," he reassured the nation, and we should not allow the cure (i.e., the shutdowns) to be worse than the disease. But in July, with sagging polls as his motivation, President Trump was again holding afternoon briefings from the White House. This time, unlike in the spring, he flew solo. His public health experts were nowhere to be seen or heard.

The briefings themselves were of little substance. The president's remarks followed a predictable pattern. Things were going well, of course, and his administration was doing a terrific job in managing the crisis. A miracle vaccine was expected and would be produced in record time, the Democrats were trying to make him look bad by resisting the reopening of schools in the fall, and the media was reporting "fake news." His daily "campaign speeches" during these briefings were predictable in their content and largely fact-free. He also reverted to form by engaging in messaging that contradicted science and his governmental experts.

The president had promoted hydroxychloroquine as a coronavirus cure during his spring briefings. The science simply did not show that this drug was a cure. Indeed, ongoing analysis had shown that it was of absolutely no use against the virus. But it was once again embraced by the president in August. Rather than accepting the evidence that it was not a cure, the president retweeted the remarks of Dr. Stella Immanuel. She had produced a video that promoted hydroxychloroquine. "You don't need masks; there is a cure," she said. "You don't need people to be locked down." The truth is that federal regulators had cited the growing evidence that hydroxychloroquine does not work as a COVID-19 cure. In addition, it was found to have deadly side effects in some cases. Furthermore, even if it had been effective as a treatment, it would not have negated the need for masks and other defensive measures to contain the outbreak of the disease.

As for Dr. Stella Immanuel, she was trained in Nigeria, and she was indeed a medical doctor. She also claimed that "spirit husbands" and "spirit wives" visited humans in their dreams and caused impotence and various gynecological problems. So here was the leader of the free world promoting a quack who states that gynecological problems are caused by sex with demons. It goes without saying that this certainly captured the media's attention. When the president was inevitably asked about Immanuel's bizarre theories, he doubled down, saying, "I thought her voice was an important voice, but I know nothing about her."[32] But fueled by the president's retweets, her ravings about the DNA of space aliens were soon flooding social media and cable news outlets. One would think that the presidential promotion of such a medical "authority" over his own scientific and public health experts would not be regarded as stable and effective leadership in a time of crisis.

The president also doubled down in his support for hydroxychloroquine as a cure. In addition to Dr. Immanuel's presidentially endorsed promotion of the "cure," legitimate debate resurfaced after the release of a study by the Henry Ford Medical Center that suggested that the drug could help mildly ill coronavirus patients recover faster. Most experts, including and especially Dr. Fauci, were quick to note that the study was flawed and that there was absolutely no evidence to suggest that hydroxychloroquine was a cure. Nevertheless, the president posted a dozen tweets in a single day in defense of the drug as a treatment. "I happen to think it works," he stated. He also continued to spend precious time in his daily coronavirus briefings promoting the drug.[33]

By the first week of August, most Americans were saying that the president was doing a poor job of managing the pandemic. Yet another survey, this one by the Pew Research Center, found that 37 percent said he was doing an excellent or good job in responding to the coronavirus outbreak, while 63 percent said he is doing only a fair or poor job. Positive views of the performance of public health officials had also declined significantly. In August, 63 percent said public health officials, such as those with the CDC, were doing an excellent or good job in responding to the coronavirus outbreak, down from 79 percent in March (see table 5.4). It should be noted that the 16 percent decline in public confidence in the public health officials came almost entirely from Republicans.

Table 5.4   Evaluating Response to Coronavirus

Percent Who Rate the Job Each of the Following Is Doing in Coronavirus Response

	Poor	Fair	Good	Excellent	Net Positive
Hospitals/medical centers	3%	9%	45%	43%	88%
Public health officials	11%	25%	47%	16%	63%
Local elected officials	12%	27%	47%	13%	60%
State elected officials	18%	26%	40%	16%	56%
President Trump	48%	15%	22%	15%	37%

Source: Pew Research Center, https://www.pewresearch.org/politics/2020/08/06/most-americans-say-state-governments-have-lifted-covid-19-restrictions-too-quickly/

As the month of August began, the debate over whether it was safe to reopen schools for the fall was heating up. The president, and many Republican governors, applied as much persuasion or pressure as they could to influence the resumption of normal face-to-face education. This was said to be best for the children and necessary to enable parents to get back to work and for the economy to reopen. President Trump even argued that children were basically immune to the virus or that it did not impact them in a life-threatening way. Assurances were given that neither students nor teachers and staff should worry. Schools could reopen safely, or so it was maintained. Ironically, just as these things were being seriously put forth by the president and others, the numbers began to tell a different story. More than ninety-seven thousand U.S. children had tested positive for the coronavirus during the last two weeks of July. According to data from the American Academy of Pediatrics and the Children's Hospital Association, that number represented more than a quarter of the number of all children diagnosed nationwide since March.[34]

During the first week of August, one Georgia high school had reopened with in-person instruction. Within a day of the reopening, photos went viral on social media showing hallways packed shoulder to shoulder with students, many of whom were not wearing masks. A week later, the newsfeeds were telling the country that this high school was temporarily reverting to virtual instruction. The school had been closed and was being cleaned after six students and three teachers tested positive for COVID19. The student who had taken and circulated the photos was briefly suspended and reported that she was facing threats from classmates.

The debates surrounding the reopening of schools, and the experiences the schools would have to endure, continued to be an important and ongoing part of the pandemic crisis as it moved into the fall. Other numbers at the beginning of August suggested a rough fall as well. On August 9, the number of coronavirus cases reported in the United States had topped five million. More than one million of these cases had been reported in just the previous seventeen days alone. The case tally in the United States had doubled since late June. The American caseload now accounted for approximately a quarter (25 percent) of all cases reported worldwide. On August 9, the worldwide numbers showed over twenty million registered cases of COVID-19 and 750,000 deaths. On August 10, the United States death toll topped 165,000. If one was looking for good news on August 9 or 10, one might have looked to New Zealand. New Zealand had just announced its one hundredth consecutive day without community transmission of the virus.[35]

Conclusion: An Unending Wave

It was October 24, 2019—forty-five days before the world's first suspected case of COVID-19 would be announced. Americans were blissfully unaware of what would soon become their living nightmare. On that date, the Johns Hopkins Center for Health Security published its Global Health Security (GHS) Index. This index consisted of research to provide a public benchmarking of health security and related capabilities across the 195 countries that make up the nations that are party to International Health Regulations. The index was a scorecard that ranked countries on how well prepared they were to respond to serious disease outbreaks (i.e., epidemics and pandemics). Nations were assessed on a range of measures, including how quickly a country was likely to respond and how well its health care system would perform. The United States ranked first out of 195 nations.[36] The United States was considered the world's best prepared nation, by this measure, for a pandemic. By early August 2020, the United States was (with over five million cases, over 165,000 deaths, and with case numbers and the death toll spiking out of control) arguably the world's biggest failure in responding to COVID-19. How in the world could this GHS Index get it so wrong? The short answer is that this index did not account for the political context in which a national policy response to a pandemic would be formulated and implemented.

Presidents George W. Bush and Barack Obama had done a great deal to advance American planning and preparedness for a major pandemic. Reflecting on the first seven months of 2020, it would appear that their planning had not been able to guarantee a successful response to a pandemic. Why? Because neither they nor their plans anticipated a Donald

Trump. Frankly, no one could have anticipated Donald Trump. We know that the outgoing Obama administration had urged the new Trump administration to continue preparedness activities for a pandemic that could be the worst since 1918. The importance of a coordinated federal response was emphasized. The Trump team reportedly dismissed this advice. Long before COVID-19 was a reality to be dealt with, President Trump and his administration had devalued the importance of public health investments and degraded the nation's pandemic preparedness capabilities. In May 2018, the Trump administration shut down the White House National Security Council directorate devoted to pandemic preparedness. It is true that the deep budget cuts Trump had proposed for the CDC and other health agencies were largely rejected by Congress, but the Trump White House did succeed in gutting the CDC's Public Health Science and Surveillance program.

In January 2020, the WHO told nations to prepare for containment, active surveillance, early detection, isolation, case management, contact tracing, and prevention of the spread of the coronavirus. The United States alone among the nations of the world seemed not to get the message, as its leader and his minions apparently believed that the United States, exceptional nation that it is, would escape the viral outbreaks that were happening in the rest of the world. Faith in American exceptionalism and wishful thinking proved to be poor substitutes for the WHO's guidance and that of American public health experts on preventing transmission of the coronavirus. What was needed, and nowhere in evidence, was a national strategy.

In the early days of the pandemic, the president was assuring us everything was under control. He assured us that travel bans would keep the virus out of the country. We only had nine cases, and then we only had fifteen cases, but he told us that it would soon be zero. As the cases mounted, the president complained that talk of a pandemic was either a hoax being promoted by his political enemies or a minor thing like the seasonal flu. In reality, we soon saw health care and case workers up to their knees in patients. Many were working in hospitals without suitable personal protective equipment (PPE) or access to testing. Nurses were forced to use trash bags to protect their bodies and bandanas instead of N95 masks.

The president left it up to the governors to deal with the minutiae of the pandemic, but he criticized those who vigorously implemented necessary restrictions to slow the spread of the disease. The president also contradicted his public health experts. He promoted hydroxychloroquine as a cure for COVID-19, even though all the legitimate research showed it was ineffective and, in some cases, dangerous. The president refused to wear a face mask and encouraged his supporters to defy stay-at-home orders. He also forced the CDC to water down or withhold scientifically sound advice and guidelines for the safe reopening of the economy in the spring and of schools in the fall. In short, it may be suggested that the best prepared nation in the world distinguished itself by simply doing next to nothing to slow the spread of the pandemic. Its years of preparation counted for naught, as all the planning and experiences of the preceding two decades would be ignored. Countries that ranked low on the GHS Index (i.e., Mongolia (46), Vietnam (50), and Iceland (58)) succeeded far beyond the best prepared nation in responding to the pandemic.[37]

It can be said that every country struggled to contain the coronavirus, and it can also be said that they made some mistakes along the way. But one country stood alone as the only affluent nation to have suffered a severe and sustained outbreak for more than four months—the United States. During the month of July, the United States had more than five times as many new cases as in all of Europe, Canada, Japan, South Korea, and Australia combined. Some countries were beginning to experience new outbreaks during this time, but these outbreaks still paled in comparison to those in the United States. The toll of the virus in the United States had, as one might suspect, fallen disproportionately on poorer people and groups that have long suffered discrimination. Black and Latino residents of the United States, according to numerous media reports, had contracted the virus at roughly three times the rate of white residents. As Americans absorbed all this information and reflected on the unthinkable conclusion that the United States was the world's greatest failure among advanced nations in controlling the spread of the virus, they could not help but ask themselves how such a thing could happen. If they understood their culture, and if they understood the politics of their time, they would have understood two central causes that might have hindered the United States in confronting a major pandemic.

The United States is a large country. This in and of itself presented some challenges that other nations may not have faced. More important may have been the nation's tradition of prioritizing individualism over all else and its reflexive resistance to government and any restrictions it might impose for the public welfare. Even in a crisis, it could be expected that Americans would chafe at the imposition of restrictions and place their individual wants and preferences over the common good. This basic component baked into the American cultural character suggests that the nation's leadership has to be exceptional and persuasive in bringing about the national unity necessary for successfully responding to a pandemic crisis. In this context, one could reasonably suggest that the poor results in the United States stemmed in substantial measure from the performance of the Trump administration.

In no other advanced nation—in very few countries at all in fact—had political leadership departed from expert advice as frequently and significantly as the Trump administration. As previously discussed, President Trump had said the virus was not a serious problem. He had predicted it would "just go away." For weeks, he questioned the need for masks; encouraged resistance to state stay-at-home orders; encouraged states to reopen quickly, even with large and growing caseloads; and routinely promoted medical disinformation. In his public appearances, from January through August, the president attempted to make the situation sound less dire than it was.

Many Republican governors followed the president's lead in downplaying the virus while ignoring the science. Democratic governors had more generally heeded scientific advice, but their performance in containing the virus was also uneven. Most governors were too quick and, in some cases, too blatantly reckless in reopening their economies. In general, governors chose to reopen before the medical experts thought it wise or safe. The desire to put people back to work and get the economy back up and running is understandable, but the rush to reopen only served to spark a huge new outbreak of the virus. The economy never benefited, and the pandemic was nowhere near under control.

The countries that had been successful in controlling the pandemic were those in which the shutdowns and closures (stay-at-home orders) had been more comprehensive than in the United States, and they had been enforced for a longer period of time. Their reopenings had also been more gradual and cautious. They had followed the science more closely, and they had had a more coherent national strategy and a well-defined strategic direction. The U.S. response to the pandemic was shaped by the national skepticism toward collective action, the Trump administration's disorganized and nonurgent response to the virus, the lack of a coherent national strategy, and fifty states moving in different directions as the varying and discordant (and too often blatantly partisan) winds blew them. The "first wave" of the COVID-19 pandemic never really ended in the United States. Its chaotic and disorganized response never brought the spread of the disease under control. It simply fueled ongoing spikes in infections over the summer. States reopened too quickly and in most cases without meeting the minimal thresholds established by the CDC for a safe reopening. Citizens quickly wearied of restrictions and caution, and they began to party in bars and private parties. Face coverings and social distancing were the topics for partisan debate, and, quite frankly, one could not help but feel that Americans just did not get it. They did not comprehend what a pandemic meant or what they needed to do about it. All of this, of course, comes back to leadership. Little, if any, effort had been made by the U.S. national leadership to pull the nation together to manage the challenges of the long-anticipated "worst pandemic since 1918."

By mid-August, the unanswered questions and the unknowns confronting Americans were raging as intensely as the virus itself. The U.S. Congress was debating a second round of relief as the economy continued to suffer and unemployment remained above 11 percent. For twenty straight weeks, the number of Americans who had lost their jobs and filed for unemployment insurance had topped one million per week. Congress was deadlocked and slow to agree on a package to provide relief. How long would it be before the much-needed relief came? The debates about reopening schools and universities were ongoing as the fall semester was soon to begin. What would the impact of reopening schools and universities be with respect to transmission of the disease? There had not been successful control of the spread of the virus over the summer. Were medical facilities adequately resupplied and prepared for what might be a "second wave" in the fall and winter? Would there in fact be a major second wave? Would a vaccine soon be available, and, if so, would it be efficiently produced and distributed? Would it be necessary to reinstitute stay-at-home orders? Would a national stay-at-home order become necessary to control the spread? What would the pandemic mean in relation to the national election in November? The answers to all these questions, and more, would unfold with the autumn leaves and the first snows.

Based on all that 2020 had brought through its first eight months, one would have been well advised to expect the unexpected. On October 24, 2019, no one would have expected that the world's best prepared nation would, by August 2020, be regarded by many to be the world's biggest failure in responding to COVID-19. This should serve to remind all that preparation is one thing and performance is another. No matter how excellent or flawed a plan, it is the human factor that frequently makes all the difference between success and failure. Despite all the planning over the previous two decades and having ample warning, the United States botched every possible opportunity to control the coronavirus in 2020. It failed despite its considerable advantages. Despite its immense resources, its biomedical might, its scientific expertise, and all its planning, the United States floundered because of the human element. Now the question on almost everyone's mind was the same. Would the floundering stop as summer turned to fall?

CHAPTER SIX

Failure Persists: The Dark Winter Approaches

You know the nearer your destination the more you're slip sliding away.
—Paul Simon

Any man can make mistakes, but only an idiot persists in his error.
—Cicero

Introduction

By August 27, the U.S. COVID-19 death toll had reached 181,791. In the previous twenty-four hours, 1,416 deaths had been added to the toll. The United States had also recorded 5,899,331 confirmed cases of COVID-19, and in the previous twenty-four hours, 49,053 cases had been added to that total. These numbers would continue to rise, of course. The news on August 27 noted that new COVID-19 cases were down about 20 percent since early August, but deaths remained alarmingly high, with 1,000 Americans a day still dying from the virus. The reports that COVID-19 cases were "down" may have been less meaningful than it was made to seem; positive tests were falling because fewer tests were actually being done. Another item in the news reported that there was a growing awareness of how the virus spreads and that more mask wearing was likely helping to curb the number of new cases. Debates surrounding the reopening of schools and universities in the fall were heating up, and both political parties held their presidential nominating conventions in largely virtual (and surrealistic) environments. As the corona summer was winding down, it was clear that the fall and winter months ahead would present a number of serious challenges to be confronted. Among these would be the accumulation of challenges not met in the preceding months that would inevitably influence the successes and the failures to come.

The first eight months of the pandemic had exposed Americans to the reality that their nation had not been prepared for a major public health emergency. It also exposed them to the reality that their national leadership was, to put it politely, inadequate to the task of managing the crisis. Sadly, the many failures that American citizens were made to endure were inevitable. A prime example of a compounding failure that would contribute to a failed response to the pandemic crisis was testing. Without adequate testing for the coronavirus, it would be nearly impossible to get an outbreak under control.

It was inevitable that testing for the new virus would be a problem. Years of underfunding and a crucial laboratory mistake led to weeks of delay and slowed testing as the virus's spread was undetected in the early weeks. The delays were only partially due to the design flaws in the early diagnostic tests developed by the Centers of Disease Control and Prevention (CDC). The CDC (as per the president's orders) would further complicate things by refusing to approve a working test developed by the World Health Organization (WHO). It also refused, at least initially, to approve those developed by local public health laboratories. Other critical shortcomings in the nation's capacity for diagnostic testing had existed long before the COVID-19 pandemic unfolded. The Biomedical Advanced Research and Development Authority, a branch of the U.S. Department of Health and Human Services (HHS), had prioritized grants for therapeutic treatments and vaccines in relation to disease outbreaks, but it had also severely underfunded the development of diagnostic testing. In addition to this, U.S. testing facilities would prove to be inadequate to the rapidly accelerating demand for testing.[1] Together, these things would contribute greatly to the inability of the United States to test early enough and widely enough to contain coronavirus outbreaks. Even when the initial flawed tests were addressed, the United States would continue to play catchup, and testing would not meet its targets to provide useful information in the most timely and efficient manner. The number of tests per day never quite reached the number needed to be optimal in containing the spread of the disease.[2]

Testing would prove to be the persistent Achilles' heel in the U.S. response. Even in the peak times in the hottest spots, there would be shortages of tests or delays in getting results. The tests were often rationed out to the very ill or to essential workers. Even as the availability of tests improved, the labs were often taking so long to get the results that they were of little use in slowing down the spread of the disease. This made it difficult to guide treatment and to guarantee the safe reopening of states as they ended their shutdowns.

In the midst of all this concern about testing, President Trump and the nation's governors were in open disagreement about what needed to be done and who needed to do it. The Trump administration insisted that there were plenty of tests that the states were not using. Governors insisted they could not do nearly enough testing without more help from the federal government. The governors were dealing with shortages in a number of components necessary for ramping up the testing (i.e., kits, chemical agents, swabs, personal protective equipment (PPE)). The federal government stubbornly refused to help. A press officer from the Federal Emergency Management Agency (FEMA) issued a statement saying that the states and hospitals could purchase what they needed "from manufacturers and distributors, as they normally do." The federal government would not use the Defense Production Act (DPA) to assist in enhancing the production or expedite the acquisition of the needed materials.[3] It is hard to justify this refusal to invoke the DPA in the middle of a historic pandemic. That would seem to have been a necessary and effective step to take. Instead, it would be a step not taken by a federal government that was apparently doing as little as it could to help the states respond to the unending wave of infection.

When states did find the equipment and materials they needed, it came at a steep price. Demand for the items exceeded supply, and prices soared. Without a national plan or system for coordinating such purchases during a crisis, states and hospitals were left to compete against each other and negotiate on their own. The lack of coordination during a crisis such as a global pandemic is, in most cases, an indication of a determination to fail. Across the world, the nations that had ramped up testing the quickest and that had the greatest success in getting ahead of the virus were those that had coordinated national plans that reduced time wasting confusion and expensive competition. National governments organized and expedited progress.

In addition to the lack of a coordinated national plan, the testing problem was further exacerbated by President Trump's treatment of testing as a political football rather than a necessary tool for stopping the spread of COVID-19. Early on, before the number of infections were out of control and contrary to the facts, he had asserted that anyone who wanted a test could get one. As the case numbers grew to alarming proportions, he actually came to see testing as a thing to be avoided. In a June 23 tweet, the president stated, "Cases are going up because we are testing far more than any other country, and ever expanding. With smaller testing we would show fewer cases." This reemphasized a point he had made earlier at a campaign rally in Tulsa, Oklahoma. His faithful supporters roared in support when he said, "Testing is a double-edged sword. When you test to that extent, you're going to find more people; you're going to find more cases. So, I said to my people, slow the testing down please."

Although testing had improved since the spring, it was still (in August) nowhere near where it should have been, and the president seemed to have no interest in improving things.[4] Instead of seeing testing as an important and necessary tool in a national effort to respond to the pandemic, he treated the testing itself as a problem and something to be deemphasized. His main concern, of course, had nothing to do with responding to or managing the crisis. He wanted to manipulate appearances so that the situation would be perceived as improving. It would serve him well at the polls to pull off such an illusion. The facts of the matter did not matter at all. There would not be fewer cases if the United States did less testing. The cases would just not be as visible, and, of course, we would not be able to monitor things in a manner that would generate the data needed to guide the decision-making as the United States sought to accomplish what it had thus far spectacularly failed to do—gain control of the virus.

By September 13, the number of Americans infected with the coronavirus had reached 6.5 million, and the American death toll had reached 195,000. On that Sunday night, President Donald Trump held a political rally in Nevada and his reelection campaign had not made any accommodations for the pandemic. The rally was held indoors with thousands of attendees crowded shoulder to shoulder and very few wearing masks. This took place despite the State of Nevada prohibiting indoor gatherings of larger than fifty people. "Tell your governor to open up your state," the president insisted as his loyal followers shouted their approval.

Many neutral observers expressed shock and criticized the president's rally as "reckless" and "selfish." The country was in the middle of a global pandemic, and here was the president ignoring all the defensive protocols and exposing his supporters to the possibility of infection and perhaps, in worst-case scenarios, death.[5] Watching the spectacle, one would never have guessed that a global pandemic was still killing hundreds of Americans every day (about one per minute, actually). And that is exactly the point.

Donald Trump's strategy had never been to manage the crisis. His strategy was to control the optics, manipulate perception, deny the crisis, blame China, blame the governors, ignore the experts, and win the 2020 election. The failures that had accumulated in the previous eight months and that would persist into the fall were all a matter of design. They were born of a conscious effort to play the crisis down and avoid any responsibility for relieving the inevitable suffering it might bring to bear on the American people.

Playing It Down: Managing the Crisis Is Not an Option

On September 15, the pandemic narrative would be altered by the release of Bob Woodward's new book, *Rage*. The book drew on hundreds of hours of interviews with firsthand witnesses and interviews with the president himself. It revealed the fundamental reason that the American response to COVID-19 was doomed to be a monumental failure. It was, as many had hypothesized, very much a failure by design.

On Tuesday, January 28, 2020, the president's national security adviser told him just how serious the mysterious new coronavirus was. Robert O'Brien advised the president that "this will be the biggest national security threat you face in your presidency."[6] Matt Pottinger, the deputy national security adviser, had been in contact with sources he had developed in China. He had asked them whether this new virus would be as serious as the SARS outbreak in 2003. His source told him it would be much worse. "Don't think SARS," he told Pottinger, "think influenza pandemic 1918."[7] Pottinger told the president that he was confident that the information he had received from his source was not speculation. It was based on hard data. It was solid.

This information would have alerted any president to the need for a coordinated plan of action, one driven by science. It would have alerted any president of the need to prepare the American people for what was to come. Yet, Donald Trump was not any president. His approach would be much different. On February 2, he was interviewed, as had become a tradition, on the Super Bowl pregame programming lineup. Most of the interview, conducted by Fox News anchor Sean Hannity, focused on the president's upcoming impeachment trial before the Senate. Toward the end of the interview, Hannity asked the president whether he was concerned about the new coronavirus. The president assured viewers that "we pretty much shut it down coming in from China."[8] President Trump reassured the public, as he would continue to do in the coming weeks, that they faced very little risk. Everything was under control, he asserted over and over.

   In an interview with Bob Woodward on March 19, President Trump said that his statements during the early weeks of the crisis, and after he had been told to expect a 1918-level pandemic, were designed to deliberately downplay the threat and not draw attention to it. "I always wanted to play it down," he said. "I still like playing it down because I don't want to create a panic."[9] The entire nation would hear this taped conversation broadcast over the news networks in September. It is worth taking a moment to reflect on this deliberate strategy to "play it down." Given that playing it down had seemingly been a constant theme and posture of the Trump administration and the incredible impact the pandemic ultimately had on the nation, one understandably must wonder what was the true motivation behind the play-it-down strategy? The president had been told how serious the threat was from the beginning. He knew what was about to happen. This was a public health crisis. He had the public health experts who could design the strategy to deal with such a threat and to communicate that strategy to the public in a manner that would enhance their preparedness for what was to come. There were fifteen years of pandemic planning in the bank to draw from if he had wanted to initiate a coherent national response to the coming crisis. Why, given all of that, did he play it down?

   With respect to Donald Trump, one might keep in mind the axiom that perception is reality. His entire life had been one of manufacturing his own reality. As a real estate tycoon (or con man?) and celebrity, he had always succeeded in persuading the media and the public (the gullible among us at least) to fall for the image of himself that he created through his ebullience, carping, bullying, and sheer insistence. He was a master of spin and a master of changing reality to his liking and to accommodate his interests and his ego. It was in his nature to shun bad coronavirus facts and numbers because they were an affront to his grand vision of himself and perhaps a trigger to his insecurities as well. He brushed bad numbers aside. He brushed science aside. He brushed the harsh reality of the pandemic aside and focused on better numbers (that were not real), exaggerated "successes," and rosy scenarios.

   The new revelations in the Woodward book did not make the president seem out of touch with reality so much as intentionally resistant to it. His efforts were aimed at creating the reality most beneficial to his interests and soothing to his ego, not at serving the American people and protecting them from the public health threat at hand. The COVID-19 pandemic was not a public health challenge to be met. For Donald Trump, the pandemic was a threat to his personal political interests and an affront to his image. He would manage the threat to himself even if it required him to mismanage the public health crisis. He would resist the reality of the crisis and resort to all of his well-tested methods to misdirect public attention away from the reality he did not like. His priority was, through any means necessary, to direct attention toward that better reality he would manufacture and market for his own benefit.

President Trump's disingenuous excuse for playing down the pandemic, "I don't want to create a panic," would have been laughable were the consequences not so deadly. From socialism to Antifa (a supposedly left-wing anti-fascist group but really more of a concept than an organized group), immigrant caravans, and more, Donald Trump had done nothing but try to create panic during his presidency. Examples abound. Ahead of the 2018 midterm elections, Trump, with the help of conservative media, tried to instill fear about a caravan of immigrants from South America coming to the United States. In doing so, he falsely portrayed the immigrants, who were coming to the United States to seek asylum, as "criminals"—even as studies have shown immigrants commit less crime than American citizens. Trailing in the polls and facing the possibility of defeat in November 2020, the president quickly took to fearmongering about the accuracy of election results. He would, without any supporting evidence, falsely claim that an increase in voting by mail (due to the pandemic) would lead to voter fraud.

Anticipating a defeat, President Trump did everything he could to cast doubt about the election results and to justify any tactics he might employ to disregard the results. As the president pushed for governors to reopen their states amid the COVID-19 pandemic, he falsely claimed that keeping states closed would lead to more suicides than deaths from the virus. Experts said there was no evidence Trump's warning of mass suicides would occur. He warned that the Green New Deal (nothing more than a concept really that was being advocated by some Democrats) to address climate change would permanently eliminate all planes, cars, cows, oil, gas, and the military. None of this was true of course. During his impeachment trial before the Senate in early 2020, President Trump warned that if he was removed from office there would almost certainly be a violent civil war. Causing panic and dividing and polarizing the country was pure Trump. And in the middle of a historic pandemic that was killing Americans, a disease much older and more difficult to tame than the new coronavirus pandemic would become a lightning rod for polarized debate and more presidentially induced panic.

On May 25, 2020, George Floyd, an unarmed Black man, died in police custody when a Minneapolis officer knelt on his neck for about eight minutes. The ghastly sight of this tragedy was filmed by an observer and broadcast across the nation. All saw what most Americans would quickly agree was the murder of a Black man by police. They heard George Floyd plead for his life and utter the words that echoed in the hearts of every civilized human being: "I can't breathe." The capturing of the final minutes of George Floyd's life on camera sparked a national outcry and demands for police reform. Nationwide protests against police violence and racial injustice surged after the killing of Floyd. Americans of all races and ages were stirred to action. Protests broke out across the nation and around the world. Americans of all races soon united behind the Black Lives Matter (BLM) movement to call for racial justice, an end to police brutality, and an end to systemic racism.

The protests were a broad public response long overdue. An analysis of these protests by the nonprofit Armed Conflict Location and Event Data Project identified more than 7,750 demonstrations across 2,400 American cities between May 26 (the day after the death of George Floyd) and August 22. Fewer than 220 of those events were marked by violence or destructive activity, and those were "largely confined to specific blocks," according to the report. "The vast majority of the demonstration events associated with the BLM movement are non-violent," the group's analysis reads. "In more than 93 percent of all demonstrations connected to the movement, demonstrators have not engaged in violence or destructive activity. Peaceful protests are reported in over 2,400 distinct locations around the country."[10]

George Floyd's killing ignited the demonstrations across the country. But the protests had also organized around other victims of police violence and systemic racism across the country. Floyd's tragic death inspired a growing number of Americans to call for justice in the tragic number of cases and other past incidents that remained unresolved. In many local communities, protests marking Floyd's death were also acts of remembrance for the too many victims of such deadly abuse of authority by law enforcement.

Despite the data indicating that the protests associated with the BLM movement were overwhelmingly peaceful, organized disinformation campaigns were quick to develop. This disinformation was aimed at spreading a deliberate mischaracterization of groups involved in the protests. One disinformation thrust sought to portray activists who support Black Lives Matter as violent extremists. Some claimed that an anti-fascist group known as Antifa was behind the protests. Antifa (more of a concept than an organized group) was said to be a terrorist organization coordinated or manipulated by hostile and external forces. All of this was pure nonsense, of course.

Many also exaggerated the violence of the BLM protests. Despite the media focus on looting and vandalism, and without dismissing the seriousness of looting and vandalism, there is little evidence to suggest that demonstrators had engaged in widespread violence. In some cases where demonstrations did turn violent, there were reports of provocateurs or infiltrators (including and especially right-wing white supremacy groups) instigating the violence.[11] And what was Donald Trump's leadership strategy as the nation grieved over the Floyd tragedy and the mounting number of such tragedies? It was predictable.

Instead of calming the nation and pointing it toward constructive steps that could be taken to address the mounting injustices and legitimate concerns, President Trump escalated the use of force against the demonstrators. He exaggerated the unrest and engaged in a wider and unnecessary push to militarize the federal government's response. He promoted the false narrative linking demonstrations to supposed left-wing groups like the fictitious Antifa, which the administration viewed as a "terrorist" organization. In an incredible display, the president used National Guard troops, Secret Service agents, and U.S. Park Police to violently disrupt a peaceful protest in Lafayette Square so that he could have a photo opportunity in front St. John's Church. Holding a book (the Bible) he had never read in front of a church he had never attended and smashing the First Amendment rights of peaceful protestors to do it was not exactly going to calm the nation. But that was not the president's goal.

President Trump next deployed federal authorities to Portland, Oregon (where protests had resulted in some violence) to keep the peace. Prior to the deployment, over 83 percent of the demonstrations in Oregon had been nonviolent. Postdeployment, the percentage of violent demonstrations rose from under 17 percent to over 42 percent, suggesting that the president's tactic had only aggravated the unrest. In the city of Portland, violent demonstrations occurred at nearly 62 percent of all events after federal agents arrived on the scene.[12] As with the pandemic, the president's response had nothing to do with addressing the nation's concerns about the problem (i.e., racial justice and police brutality). It was about creating a different reality to fit the narrative that he wanted to use in his reelection campaign. He would be the "law and order" candidate. Only he, the president's political ads and stump speeches would remind the nation, could protect Americans against protesters who were, by his fanciful reckoning, lawless and radical socialists bent on destroying their businesses and neighborhoods.

There are many more examples one could cite of President Trump's efforts to misdirect the American public with manufactured realities in the constant effort to promote his own interests. The only thing that mattered to Donald Trump was Donald Trump. Dr. Anthony Fauci noted, according to Bob Woodward's book, that throughout the entire coronavirus pandemic, the only thing that mattered to Donald Trump was his reelection. Politics and the personal interests of Donald Trump were the only things that mattered in the administration's response to the pandemic.[13] This puts the dizzying insanity of the American response to COVID-19 in perspective. At every key moment of decision, the interests of Donald Trump required the prioritization of politics (more precisely Trumpian politics) over science. A quick reminder of what 2020 and the president's response to date had shown the nation by the fall of 2020 serves to emphasize this conclusion.

From the beginning, as we have seen and as Bob Woodward would confirm, President Trump publicly played down the virus, even though he privately acknowledged that he knew the seriousness of the threat. As the virus began spreading across the country, the president was bent on minimizing the dangers. Instead of developing and implementing a national strategy to address the threat, the president accelerated the polarization of the country. The simple acts of wearing a mask and social distancing to control the spread of the virus became political wedge issues because of doubt sown by the president. Even as the hospitals in New York City were deluged with patients and the bodies of the dead were stored in refrigerated trucks, the president refused to prepare the rest of the nation for what was coming its way. "It will go away" was the totality and the substance of his response.

As the death chart began to explode across the country, the president criticized state governors for their science-driven stay-at-home orders. He contradicted his White House coronavirus response coordinator, Dr. Anthony Fauci, and other experts who advised that unless the country adopted masks, practiced social distancing, and kept businesses closed, the death toll could not be slowed. Instead of issuing a national mask mandate and other recommended measures, the Trump administration pushed for a quick reopening of the economy. The president's stated rationale was that the cure was worse than the disease. As the states reopened, the predictable happened. Cases surged, and the death toll mounted.

As the death toll rose, the president refused to wear a mask in public, continued his public rallies where masks were not required and social distancing was ignored, downplayed all CDC data tracking the disease, and continued to justify a quick and total reopening. Eager to find a miracle cure, the president promoted hydroxychloroquine (an antimalarial drug) as a "game changer," despite the scientific evidence that there was no proof that the drug was effective as a treatment and experts warning that it might be dangerous. Later in the summer, and again without scientific proof, the president promoted convalescent plasma as a treatment. Clearly, science was not a weapon Donald Trump wished to employ in battling the COVID-19 pandemic. In fact, he spent inordinate time and effort trying to discredit science. Why? Because he did not think the reality portrayed by science would help him in his quest for reelection.

Rejecting the advice of scientific experts appealed to the president and his followers. Such irrationality set well with the president's political image as an outsider. He had cultivated the image of being the scourge of the elite political, academic, and scientific establishments. This was part of a strategy to solidify his bond with his supporters, most of whom prized that image and who themselves shared Trump's reluctance to accept any educated elite or scientific expertise that might contradict their values or beliefs.

Refusing to accept the scientific advice that may have contained the spread of COVID-19, the president and his administration routinely dismissed expert assessments of the gravity of the pandemic and refused to take the measures necessary to bring it under control. When the experts proved to be right, it became a political necessity to muzzle the scientists who contradicted the administration's alternate reality and its rosy perspective. CDC officials (current and former) "described a workforce that has seen its expertise questioned, its findings overturned for political purposes and its effectiveness in combating the pandemic undermined by partisan actors in Washington."[14] In August, a directive from HHS issued guidance recommending that those who came into contact with someone infected by the virus be tested even if they were asymptomatic. The White House removed this guidance from the CDC website. The recommendation was reinstated after a public outcry.[15] Nevertheless, ongoing political interference with the communications of the scientific agencies would have the impact of reducing public trust in them. In September, CDC Director Robert Redfield testified before Congress and said that a vaccine would not be widely available until 2021. President Trump criticized Redfield and promised that a vaccine would be ready soon, perhaps even before the election in November. This contradiction of the CDC director raised concerns over whether the public would accept a vaccine once it became available. Public confidence was not the issue for the president, and science was not the issue. The issue was his need to invent a better reality to improve his political fortunes.

President Trump did not like the scientific contradictions to his manufactured reality. Naturally, his solution was to suppress the science and control the message. As one example of this, he appointed Michael Caputo to head up communications for HHS. HHS oversees the CDC and the Federal Drug Administration. Caputo was not a scientist. He had absolutely no science background. He was a public relations consultant whose company had been hired by the Russian energy giant Gazprom. His assignment there had been to improve Russian President Vladimir Putin's image in the United States. His assignment at HHS would be to improve the communication of the president's manufactured reality, even if this meant discrediting the science and the nation's public health experts. Improving Donald Trump's image would be priority one.

President Trump's efforts to construct an alternate reality also inevitably tested his patience with Dr. Anthony Fauci and Dr. Deborah Birx and their work on the White House Coronavirus Task Force. As we have seen, by late summer, they were no longer visible to the public at the president's daily COVID press briefings. Indeed, a new "expert" was added to the task force and soon became the medical expert at the president's right hand. Dr. Scott Atlas was the newest addition to the White House Coronavirus Task Force and, most importantly, one who agreed with many of President Donald Trump's views, including the need to open all schools nationally in the fall. Atlas was a frequent Fox News guest who echoed many of Trump's beliefs about COVID-19. He had criticized the state stay-at-home orders, been a consistent voice downplaying the coronavirus pandemic, and supported the reopening of the economy and schools. He would echo the president's views perfectly. Atlas argued that children "have extremely low risk" when it comes to coronavirus, much less than the seasonal flu. Thus, it stood to reason that schools could be reopened. He also stated that he believed children were unlikely to spread the virus to adults and teachers.[16]

Of course, virtually everything Atlas said or believed was disputed by the public health experts. It should be noted that Atlas, a fellow at Stanford University's Hoover Institute, was not a public health or infectious disease specialist. This did not matter to the president because Atlas would, unlike Drs. Fauci and Birx, support the president's preferred reality 100 percent. On September 28, CDC Director Robert Redfield expressed his concern about the president's newest task force member by telling a television reporter, "Everything he says is false."[17]

Given the understood priorities of the president and the administration's track record over the preceding months, there would be no hope for managing the COVID-19 crisis any better in the fall than there had been in the spring or summer. Whatever the fall would bring, managing the crisis was not an option. On September 24, the number of confirmed cases in the United States had surpassed the seven million mark. The death toll stood at 205,614. Things were not about to improve.

America Gets Schooled

As the summer approached its midpoint, parents, administrators, doctors, and state and local politicians debated about what the best course for American schoolchildren would be amid the continuing COVID-19 pandemic. President Trump insisted that schools reopen for in-person education in the fall of 2020. In addition to putting the pandemic and its fallout on his political fortunes behind him, he felt this to be important to his goal of reopening the nation and the economy in time to boost his reelection chances. He accused those who disagreed with him about reopening the schools as having political motives. He suggested that keeping the schools closed was aimed at seeking to harm him politically. The president went so far as to tweet a threat to withhold federal funds from schools that did not open for face-to-face instruction. As this discussion heated up, and despite the reasonable desire to find a way to safely reopen the nation's schools, it needed to be understood that the reopening of schools would bring some increased risk of exposing not just students but also teachers and staff to a highly dangerous virus. Just how much risk was, as yet, unknown. There also seemed to be very little direction coming from the federal government to help the kids learn and the teachers teach while mitigating the COVID-19 risks.

As the coronavirus spread around the country in March and April, schools closed in all fifty states. Most stayed closed through the end of the academic year. These closures were, of course, meant to help slow transmission of the virus, which had already sickened parents, teachers, staff, and students nationwide. Most school districts switched to presenting instruction online. As the nation would quickly discover, delivering instruction online was a process that posed its own challenges. For example, experts worried about how the nearly one in five children who lacked a computer at home would complete remote schoolwork and how homeless students would find a place to study. The shift to remote learning also placed enormous strain on parents, who were now expected to take over as part-time educators. In addition to the burdens of working from home, where that was possible, they would now be assisting their children to complete their schoolwork from home.

It was generally agreed within the education community of experts that online instruction was inferior to face-to-face instruction, at least insofar as the needs of young schoolchildren were concerned. School psychologists also worried that students' mental health could suffer with the shift to remote schooling, especially given the added stress of the pandemic. It was felt that the problems associated with remote learning made it essential that a way be found to reopen the schools in the fall, assuming of course that this could be done safely. A failure to reopen, it was feared, would set students back further, especially those who were already marginalized within the education system and society as a whole (e.g., low-income students).

Some school districts decided to remain online or virtual through the fall semester. This was especially true in areas where the infection rate was on the climb. Many schools, especially in the nation's largest school districts and those in areas where outbreaks were spiking, chose to follow a hybrid model of in-person and virtual instruction. This included in-person learning on a staggered schedule, with students attending school two or three days per week. Such a schedule allowed for social distancing in the classroom. The wearing of masks and other safety protocols would be required in most cases. Despite these adjustments and the best efforts to implement them, some schools had to close (at least briefly) when coronavirus outbreaks occurred in the fall.

Universities also struggled with the question of reopening. Like the nation's schools, universities had also closed down and instituted remote or online learning practices as the coronavirus swept the nation in the spring of 2020. As they looked toward the fall semester, administrators and faculty debated the options before them. The struggle to salvage some normalcy and understandable concerns about their revenue flow inclined most college administrators to find a way to invite students back into dorms and classrooms. Universities are, of course, risk averse. They are also consumer oriented. Most administrators were undoubtedly torn between the desire to keep students happy, the need to keep students safe, and the need they felt to protect their revenue stream. The options being discussed were fairly obvious. Universities could continue to offer online instruction only, they could offer a hybrid of online and in-person instruction, or they could fully return to in-person instruction. By August 26, according to the *New York Times*, the tracking of plans for some three thousand institutions revealed that only 20 percent of the nation's universities would resume primarily in-person instruction. Twenty-seven percent would remain primarily online and 6 percent online only. Fifteen percent would opt for a hybrid of online and in-person classes, and 6 percent were doing something else entirely.[18]

All universities that resumed some on-campus, in-person, or hybrid options did so with what were felt to be sufficiently strict rules in place. These included no parties, regular coronavirus tests, the wearing of masks, social distancing, self-reporting of symptoms, and mandatory quarantines. The prospect of filling up campus dorms, classrooms, and cafeterias with students presented numerous threats to be managed during a global pandemic.

Most universities that resumed in-person or hybrid models implemented a number of strategies designed to prevent the spread of the virus. Some required mandatory testing of all students, faculty, and staff as they arrived for the beginning of the semester. Classrooms and cafeterias were reconfigured to maintain appropriate social distancing. The wearing of face masks was mandatory. Many universities minimized class sizes and staggered attendance by combining in-person and virtual techniques. Campuses struggled to develop detailed and properly resourced plans for tracing and quarantine. They also beefed up their PPE supplies and staffing for infirmaries.

Students would be discouraged from going home or traveling during the semester. It was also suggested that all public gatherings, concerts, plays, sporting events, and social activities be canceled. Finally, universities needed to be prepared to close the campus and revert to an online format should an anticipated fall wave occur or changing circumstances on a campus dictate. Despite all these adjustments to reopen the campuses "safely," students became infected, universities rebuked them for it, and some campuses inevitably closed back down.

Shortly after the beginning of classes, coronavirus cases spiked almost immediately at the University of North Carolina at Chapel Hill and Notre Dame. These outbreaks were linked to large student parties. Both schools shut down in-person education and switched to online-only classes. Within a few days of reopening, Syracuse University suspended twenty-three people after a large outdoor gathering. Officials expressed the concern that this gathering could have done enough damage to shut down campus, including residence halls and in-person learning, before the academic semester even began.[19] From the very outset of the new semester, almost every campus experienced some coronavirus spread and some disruption due to the quarantining of students or faculty or staff. This was, of course, an inevitability when dealing with a highly contagious virus.

The concerns that seemed to motivate the planning and the preparations universities had undertaken to prepare for anything but a normal fall semester focused on priorities well beyond the highly contagious virus. Universities were facing intense political and financial pressure to bring in tuition and other revenues to offset their costs. Students were concerned about getting their money's worth (i.e., getting what their tuition was supposed to pay for). Idealistic educators were concerned about optimal teaching environments. In this mix of concerns, one could not help but wonder where the biological and moral realities of a deadly pandemic were factored into the decisions that were made. Some cynics wondered whether universities were pulling a fast one. In a tweet at the beginning of the fall semester, Nate Silver put it bluntly: "What some colleges are doing isn't so far from a bait-and-switch. Lay out implausible conditions under which college could commence w/o COVID spread. Get tuition on premise of an in-person experience. Blame students when the conditions are inevitably violated. Then go online."[20] It was at least reasonable to wonder whether the return to in-person instruction might have been motivated by a misreading of scientific probabilities and a flawed balancing of interests. Was it possible that the weighting of economic harms and optimal teaching environments had improperly tipped the balance away from the public health impacts that needed to be addressed as a first priority?

Most universities seemed determined to forge ahead despite any warning signs. Many Division I college football teams proceeded to go ahead with their seasons even as games were canceled or postponed due to coronavirus outbreaks among players, coaches, and staff. Tensions over outbreaks on campuses inevitably boiled over in some college towns. The University of Wisconsin–Madison saw over twenty-eight hundred confirmed cases by the end of September. This caused the campus to close down in-person instruction for two weeks. Local government officials demanded that the university send every student home. The university refused to do so. Rhode Island's Democratic governor, Gina Raimondo, complained that outbreaks on two campuses had boosted the state's infection rate high enough to put it on the list of places whose residents were required to quarantine when traveling to New York. Some universities were more successful than others, impressively so in some cases, but the fact remained that thousands of college students around the country were quarantined in their dorm rooms or apartments.

Between the beginning of the fall semester on the nation's university campuses and October 8, there were more than 178,000 COVID-19 cases and 70 coronavirus-related deaths on some fourteen hundred college campuses across the United States.[21] Most universities employed the recommended evidence-based measures to fight the virus. These included social distancing, testing, tracing, and isolating. But both the implementation and the success of these measures in combating outbreaks varied widely from campus to campus. At some schools, all students had to get tested at least once a week if they wanted to remain on campus. At others, even students with COVID-19 symptoms had difficulty getting tested at all.

Some schools provided single-occupancy rooms for students who should quarantine after being exposed to the virus. Others sent students back to their dorms to wait to see whether they got sick.[22] It is little wonder that some students were soon heard to complain about being made to come back to campus and compromise their safety so that their university could make money. They also complained that they were not getting a "discount" as many of their classes were online and many amenities were shut down.

With respect to the nation's schools, by October 1, the nation began to have a sense of how common COVID-19 was in schools that had reopened and what schools were doing to reduce the spread of the virus. Infection rates among teachers and staff were markedly higher than those among students. This was not a surprise given previous evidence that suggested adults were more likely to contract the virus. Even the hybrid models employed by many districts to make schools safer did not eliminate the risks of infection. While there was a need for more data to draw significant conclusions on the risks to students, teachers, staff, and the broader community, a picture was beginning to emerge.

The approaches to education during a pandemic were widely varied. California, for example, had issued guidelines barring districts from opening if transmission was too high. Others, like Florida, pressured all schools to open regardless of transmission rates. In some states, decisions were left up to the individual districts themselves. Efforts to map reopening around the country looked like a confusing patchwork of quilts. Almost half the school districts across the United States had planned to start the school year fully in person. Rural districts were the most likely to plan a fully in-person start, with 65 percent indicating such a plan. This compared with 24 percent of suburban districts and 9 percent of urban ones. Nearly four out of five urban districts planned to start the year fully remote.[23] Whatever they had planned, schools were constantly changing their plans in the face of changing viral conditions or various political pressures.

Even by mid-October, it was unclear how many K–12 schools had fully reopened. This was due to the country's sprawling network of school districts, each under varying levels of state and local control. As reported in *Education Week*, four states had ordered all schools to reopen. Seven states, along with Washington, DC, and Puerto Rico, mandated partial or full closures. The remaining thirty-nine states had by and large left it up to individual school districts or local governments to decide based on local conditions.[24]

There did not seem to have been a massive surge of COVID-19 due to K–12 schools reopening for in-person instruction. Confirmed cases in

K–12 schools made up less than 2 percent of all cases reported in the United States between August and mid-October.[25] But many states and school districts were not reporting COVID-19 cases in K–12 schools. In addition to incomplete data, there were many unknowns about how much children, especially younger children, might spread the coronavirus. Experts had confirmed that adolescents ages twelve to seventeen were roughly twice as likely as children ages five to eleven years old to have a confirmed coronavirus infection. Whether that meant younger children were less likely to get and transmit the coronavirus or merely less likely to develop significant symptoms was still an open question.

As of October 15, there had been fifty-two thousand confirmed cases of COVID-19 in K–12 schools. While not an insignificant number, it was generally concluded that reopening the schools had not led to an explosion of cases as some had feared.[26] It bears noting that more than 277,000 children, ages five to seventeen, were confirmed infected between March and September 19, with an increase in September after a peak and a decline over the summer. The numbers may have actually been higher given that testing was most often done on people with symptoms, and children with the coronavirus often have no symptoms. It should also be noted that weekly COVID-19 cases among people ages eighteen to twenty-two increased 55 percent nationally. These increases were greatest in the Northeast and Midwest and were not solely attributable to increased testing. By October 1, children of all ages made up 10 percent of all U.S cases, up from 2 percent in April.[27] Most infected children were seen to have mild cases, and hospitalizations and death rates were much lower than in adults.

While the nation had not yet seen the types of coronavirus outbreaks that would force most school districts that had reopened to close back down, the communities in which schools had aggressively reopened did experience an alarming new wave of cases. By October, these new waves were especially alarming across the upper Midwest. Whether this was a price paid for aggressively reopening schools or merely the result of increased community spread, it was nevertheless interesting to see that communities that had been aggressive about reopening would experience an alarming increase in coronavirus cases in the fall. While reopened schools were generally seeing lower infection rates than their surrounding communities, there was more that remained unknown than was definitively known about the impact of reopening the schools. It was also very unclear which policies were most effective at curbing the spread of the disease in schools. Not all schools reported statistics the same way, and every district had its own set of reopening guidelines.[28] It was pretty clear that everyone was making it up as they went along.

The lack of national leadership and a national strategy once again left the nation running in different directions from state to state and school district to school district. As always, events would overtake a disorganized nation. In October, a two-week uptick in COVID-19 cases among children underscored just how much still needed to be learned. According to the American Academy of Pediatrics and the Children's Hospital Association, there had been a 13 percent increase in child cases reported from September 24 to October 8. More than seventy-seven thousand new COVID cases in children had been reported during this two-week period.[29]

As October moved toward November, the entire nation would be "schooled" again as a predicted fall wave brought a dramatic surge in COVID-19 cases. It was quickly evident that the fall wave could overwhelm hospitals, kill thousands of Americans a day by January, and leave even young survivors with long-term complications. The fall/winter surge that experts had warned about and that everyone with a clue had been worried about was now happening, especially in the northern Midwest, where state after state was getting hit very hard. It would soon be a national wave. By mid-October, thirty states were reporting alarming new spikes in cases, according to data from Johns Hopkins University.[30] The nation was, as President Trump would suggest, "rounding the corner." But what was around that corner was not anything that would be welcomed by anyone. The nation's "schooling" was just beginning.

Rounding the Corner or Running in Circles?

The U.S. president announced in the small hours of October 2, 2020, that he and First Lady Melania Trump would be going into quarantine after they were both found to have contracted the dreaded coronavirus. The president, who had flouted social distancing guidelines and ridiculed mask wearing while drawing thousands to tightly packed campaign events, had never abided by any of the recommended protocols for slowing the spread of the virus. Just two days before, on September 30, President Trump had held a rally in Minnesota that drew thousands, contravening social distancing guidelines and local officials who warned that the state was already experiencing "uncontrolled spread" of the virus due to large outdoor gatherings. One day later, and after being told that senior adviser Hope Hicks (who had traveled with him to Minnesota on Air Force One) had tested positive, the president could have exposed scores of people to COVID-19 after appearing symptomatic at a fundraiser at his New Jersey golf club and not wearing a mask. Now, ironically, the president himself had contracted the virus.

The president would have access to world-class and taxpayer-funded health care and rapid testing. This he would have even though he and Senate Republicans had blocked billions of dollars in funding for such programs for the general public. They had made gutting the Affordable Care Act enacted during the Obama administration, which had expanded health care coverage for millions of Americans, a top priority. The nation watched on live television as a helicopter (Marine One) took the president from the White House to the Walter Reed National Military Medical Center, where he would receive around-the-clock treatment by a team of physicians.

Fortunately, the president's infection was a mild case. He was released from the hospital after just three short days. Before leaving the hospital, the president tweeted that he was "feeling really good." He also suggested that this coronavirus thing was no big deal. "Don't be afraid of COVID," Trump tweeted. "Don't let it dominate your life."[31] In a matter of days, the president resumed his hectic schedule of large rallies as he focused on his campaigning for the fast approaching election that would decide his future. He almost defiantly passed up an opportunity to reset his message and show solidarity with Americans who had suffered during the pandemic. Far from being chastened by his bout with COVID-19, the president returned to minimizing the danger from a pandemic that had already killed more than 210,000 of his fellow Americans. Instead, he called on supporters to not be afraid of COVID and to "get out there."[32]

There had been some speculation that a White House Rose Garden event honoring the president's new Supreme Court nominee, Amy Coney Barrett, may have been a super-spreader occasion. The attendees were not wearing masks, and, of course, social distancing protocols were not observed. Shortly after that event, a number of participants, including the president, tested positive for coronavirus. The president resumed campaigning after his short hospital stay. He was determined, or so it seemed, to hold what could only be called more super-spreader events. These events were large-scale rallies of unmasked, non-socially distanced supporters yelling in each other's faces while their "heroic" leader emitted a nonstop barrage of falsehoods, exaggerations, and barefaced lies. He repeatedly claimed that the United States was "rounding the corner" on the pandemic and that things were improving rapidly. He predicted that the evil "fake news" media would quit reporting COVID-19 fatalities come November 4 (i.e., the day after the election). He even sunk so low as to claim that health officials were motivated by greed. He falsely told his cheering crowds that the doctors and hospitals got more money if they reported that COVID-19 was the cause of death.

In Janesville, Wisconsin, on October 17, the president regaled his audience with a torrent of lies. The *New York Times* did a thorough fact-check of this particular speech. Fact-checkers documented 131 false statements during Trump's eighty-seven minutes onstage. Nearly three-quarters of everything he said was untrue. The most egregious untruths (i.e., lies) concerned COVID-19, probably because he knew that the disease represented his single greatest failure and the most damaging threat to his reelection hopes. Within the first two minutes of his speech, the president made an absurd claim: "When you look at our numbers compared to what's going on in Europe and other places, we're doing well."[33] However, the truth of the matter was quite to the contrary. The United States had more cases and deaths per capita than any major country in Europe but Spain and Belgium. The United States had just 4 percent of the world's population but accounted for 20 percent of the global deaths from COVID-19.

Despite the president's rosy assertion that we had "rounded the corner" and the White House's ridiculous contention that the president's accomplishments during his term of office included ending the pandemic, late October and early November saw a record number of new cases in the United States. In the week of October 23–30, 540,035 new COVID-19 cases were reported across the nation. This was the most for any seven-day period since July. On Friday, October 30, 98,583 new infections were reported. This was a record number of COVID cases in a single day. On that same day, 978 COVID deaths were also recorded, also a record.[34]

On November 2, the day before the 2020 election, the CDC COVID Data Tracker reported that the United States had reached 9,182,628 cases, and 565,607 of these cases had been reported in just the previous seven days. The COVID death toll in the United States had reached 230,383. Cases were increasing in most every state, with Illinois, Texas, Wisconsin, California, Florida, and Michigan leading the way.[35] The stark reality of the rapidly accelerating fall wave had overtaken the rosy presidential scenario that we had rounded a corner and the virus would soon disappear. A Harris survey conducted in the days before the election found that 66 percent of Americans feared that the worst of the COVID-19 pandemic was still to come, and 52 percent said that the pandemic was worse than they had expected it would be. Nearly four out of five (79 percent) Americans were concerned about the rise in cases of COVID-19, and more than four out of five (82 percent) were concerned that the death toll would rise past 250,000. A growing number of Americans (75 percent) were concerned about a possible shortage of health care workers, especially in states seeing an alarming and dangerous level of hospitalizations. On the weekend before the election, 69 percent of Americans indicated they were staying home as much as possible.[36] Faith in our national leaders was dwindling as the country faced a dramatic new wave of infections, and there was a growing sense that no action was being taken to slow the spread. As if to underscore the growing concern across the nation, the week after the election, the number of COVID-19 cases in the United States (which stood at 9,182,628 the day before the election) topped 10 million.

Even as public concern about the rise in new infections increased, there remained partisan differences in public perceptions. Not surprisingly, the president's supporters were less concerned about the pandemic, as they were more likely to drink the Kool-Aid he was serving up. A Pew Research Center survey conducted in the first two weeks of October showed that only 24 percent of Trump supporters viewed the coronavirus outbreak as a "very important" voting issue. Democrats and Republicans differed widely on the importance of several issues (see table 6.1), but none more so than the pandemic and the president's response to it.

Over eight in ten supporters of the Democratic nominee, former vice president Joe Biden, said the coronavirus was very important to their vote, compared with just 24 percent of Trump supporters. Since early August, the percentage of Trump voters who viewed the coronavirus as very important had declined by 15 percent. This undoubtedly corresponded to the president's strategy to put the pandemic in his rearview mirror and to essentially run away from the virus. Joe Biden had conducted his campaign in a manner that incorporated all the recommended safety and public health protocols. He did not hold large rallies that packed people together, and his campaign found creative ways (e.g., parking lot gatherings with people beeping horns for the applause lines) to keep supporters safe and maintain social distancing. Overall, a large majority of Americans disapproved of President Trump's handling of the pandemic as Election Day neared (see table 6.2), but there were predictable partisan differences, as most Republicans approved of the president's handling of the crisis.

While most Republicans considered the president's response to the pandemic appropriate, most Democrats and independents said he did not treat the virus seriously enough. This indicated, despite anyone's opinion about his response to the pandemic, that the president had succeeded in accomplishing the one thing that should never happen during a pandemic or any other public health crisis—he had made it a partisan issue.

At a time when a coherent national strategy was required and expert and precise communication mattered most (i.e., during a major public

Table 6.1　Voters Ranking of Issues Importance

Trump and Biden supporters were asked to identify which of the following issues were important to them

Issue	Biden/Lean Biden	Trump/Lean Trump	All Voters
Economy	66%	84%	74%
Health care	82%	42%	65%
Coronavirus outbreak	82%	24%	55%
Foreign policy	50%	53%	51%
Abortion	42%	48%	54%

Source: Pew Research Center, https://www.pewresearch.org/fact-tank/2020/10/21 /only-24-of-trump-supporters-view-the-coronavirus-outbreak-as-a-very-important -voting-issue/

Table 6.2　Public Evaluation of President Trump's Handling of Pandemic

Do you approve or disapprove of how Donald Trump is handling the coronavirus outbreak?

	Approve	Disapprove
All voters	35%	66%
Republicans	71%	28%
Independents	35%	62%
Democrats	9%	91%

Source: AP/NORC survey, October 8–12, 2020, https://apnorc.org/projects/concern -about-trumps-handling-of-the-pandemic-persist/

health crisis), the president had produced chaos and conflict. Under his "leadership," a near civil war erupted between the masked and the unmasked. The "lock-downers" and the "open-uppers" were having a pitched battle. The president spent much of his time during the crisis deriding experts and ignoring their scientific advice. He minimized the threat of COVID-19, even to the point of endangering his own life and the lives of those around him. Many Americans were rightly upset that their country, with only 4 percent of the world's population, had suffered 20 percent of the world's deaths. Other Americans, those who listened to and believed the president, were upset that the experts (and reality) disagreed with their leader.

Handled properly, the COVID-19 pandemic should have been a time for all Americans to come together to address a common threat. Instead, it became just another political football as the country descended into deeper acrimony. The COVID-19 virus is nonpartisan, but it will probably be long remembered for the partisan divisions it sowed among the American people in a time of crisis. Rather than gaining the ability to contain the virus, the United States was seemingly mired in a dizzying cycle of chaos and confusion, in no small measure because of the president's failed leadership. Rounding a corner always seemed to mean compounding the division and the confusion when progress was most needed but always tragically lacking.

The Economic Consequences

On April 27, 2020, President Trump stood near a sign that read, "Opening up America again." He announced his plan to reopen the nation's economy in the face of the mounting coronavirus epidemic. "Every day it gets better," he proclaimed. "We are continuing to rapidly expand our capacity and confident that we have enough testing to begin reopening and the reopening process. We want to get our country open."[37] On that day, as the president spoke, the number of confirmed cases of COVID-19 was near one million and about 55,000 people had died. By November 9, there would be over ten million cases and almost 240,000 deaths.

The efforts by the president and the states to reopen the economy were largely unsuccessful in economic terms. They were also a disaster in terms of the pandemic. As a result, in addition to millions of Americans agonizing over the course of the pandemic, some more basic concerns were also exacerbated. A growing number found themselves agonizing over whether they would have enough money to pay the rent or put food on the table. The Labor Department reported on November 5 that twenty-two million Americans were still applying for unemployment.[38] That was, by any definition, crisis-level unemployment. The federal weekly supplement to state-level benefits of $600 per week had expired in July. Two remaining programs to expand federal unemployment benefits were set to expire in December. Many Americans had already exhausted their unemployment benefits in the two remaining programs.

On November 6, a report by the Congressional Research Service provided an update of unemployment rates during the COVID-19 pandemic (see box 6.1). After a sharp rise in unemployment beginning in February and March, unemployment peaked at unprecedented numbers by April. By October, the country was able to add back a number of jobs as the economy reopened across the nation. But this was not the quick V-shaped recovery that optimists had predicted. Many jobs had not come back. By

October and November, the pace of rehiring had slowed dramatically. It was not nearly robust enough to bring the economy back to "normal." Even with the rehiring that had occurred, the economy remained more than ten million jobs in the hole. Experts were saying that at the pace things were going, it would be two years or more before the United State recovered all the jobs lost since February 2020.[39]

The recovery, such as it was, was more of a K-shaped recovery. The well-to-do and the professional strata had seen improvement, but most of

---

Box 6.1   Unemployment Rates during the COVID-19 Pandemic: In Brief

- The unemployment rate peaked at an unprecedented level, not seen since data collection started in 1948, in April 2020 (14.7 percent) before declining to a still-elevated level in October (6.9 percent).

- In April, every state and the District of Columbia reached unemployment rates greater than their highest unemployment rates during the Great Recession.

- Unemployment is concentrated in industries that provide in-person services. Notably, the leisure and hospitality industry experienced an unemployment rate of 39.3 percent in April, before declining to 16.3 percent in October.

- Part-time workers experienced an unemployment rate almost twice that of their full-time counterparts in April (24.5 percent vs. 12.9 percent), but this gap has since closed.

- Workers without a college degree experienced worse unemployment rates in April (e.g., 21.2 percent for workers with no high school degree) than workers with a bachelor's degree or higher (8.4 percent). The gap between educated and less-educated workers remained in October.

- Teenaged women experienced an unemployment rate of 36.6 percent in April, and teenaged men, 28.6 percent; compared with 13.7 percent for women and 12.1 percent for men ages 25–54. The gap between men and women has since narrowed overall, but young workers are still experiencing relatively high rates of unemployment.

- Racial and ethnic minorities had relatively high unemployment rates in April (16.7 percent for Black workers compared to 14.2 percent for White workers, and 18.9 percent for Hispanic workers compared to 13.6 percent for non-Hispanic workers), and these gaps persisted in October.

Source: Congressional Research Service, https://crsreports.congress.gov/product/pdf/R/R46554

the rest of the workforce, especially the less educated, saw things continue to worsen. As the expected fall spike in new coronavirus infections took off, it was clear that the industries that had suffered the most job losses (i.e., travel, leisure, and hospitality) would be in for a very long and difficult winter. There were many reasons to suspect that the robust fall wave would decelerate the rate at which jobs in general would be recovered in the coming months.

Dr. Anthony Fauci, the nation's top infectious disease expert, was absolutely correct when he noted in April that "unless we get the virus under control, the real recovery economically is not going happen." He was spot-on when he added, "So what you do if you jump the gun and go into a situation where you have a big spike (in more coronavirus cases), you're going to set yourself back."[40]

The rush to reopen the American economy produced two very different outcomes. It was great for Wall Street, where stocks soared over the summer as companies closed a striking $496 billion in mergers and acquisitions. Meanwhile, ten million cases and over 240,000 deaths by early November as well as ten million jobs in the hole suggested that the rest of the country and the economy in general were in big trouble. Main Street was still waiting for help, and millions of families and small businesses were in economic distress. Despite the push to quickly reopen the economy after the spring shutdowns, the economy faltered as the nation debated the use of masks and social distancing and predictably failed to stem the tide of coronavirus infections. Economists stressed that the course of the virus would dictate the course of the economy—and that the United States was still very far from being back to business as usual. Help was needed, but it did not seem to be on the way.

The March Coronavirus Relief Act, known as the CARES Act, was a $2 trillion aid package that provided financial assistance to families and businesses impacted by COVID-19. By May, it became clear that more help was needed to respond to the economic wreckage brought on by the pandemic. The Democratic-controlled U.S. House of Representatives approved another coronavirus relief package in mid-May. This legislation, known as the HEROES Act, would have provided funds for state and local governments, hazard pay for frontline workers, expanded paid leave benefits, and student loan debt forgiveness. The Republican-controlled U.S. Senate sat on the legislation and simply refused to bring it up for a vote.

The HEROES Act that was passed by the House included specific provisions that would have addressed concerns in the workplace. More nonprofits would be eligible for Paycheck Protection Program (PPP) loans, and it offered relief to more struggling small businesses that kept workers on payroll during the pandemic. Another feature would allow employers to use PPP loans for longer than the currently approved eight-week period. They would also have until December 3 (rather than June 30) under the loan forgiveness rules to rehire laid off workers. More funds would also be made available to small businesses through the Economic Injury Disaster Loan program. Under the HEROES Act, employers would have been reimbursed by the federal government for offering hazard and incentive pay to essential workers. The federal government's $600 weekly supplement to state unemployment benefits (provided for in the CARES Act) would continue until January 31, 2021. The extra unemployment payments were otherwise set to expire on July 31. But, as noted, the Republican Senate refused to even bring up the HEROES Act for a vote once it had passed the House (along party lines). The HEROES Act would also have provided $500 billion in direct assistance to state governments to counter the fiscal impacts of the pandemic as well as $375 billion to assist local governments, $20 billion to tribal governments, and $20 billion to U.S. territories.[41]

The HEROES Act was dead on arrival in the Senate. Republicans were said to be appalled by the $3 trillion price tag. President Trump threatened to veto the bill if it passed the Senate. Senate Republicans would simply not bring it up for a vote, saying the measure was a "liberal wish list" that included many provisions entirely unrelated to the current economic crisis.[42] Between the months of May and November, Republican and Democratic congressional leaders could not agree on a second coronavirus stimulus relief bill. President Trump also frustrated any negotiations to arrive at a compromise by constantly shifting his position on what, if any, stimulus was needed.

The refusal of Democrats and Republicans to cooperate with one another was not unexpected. Just as they held differing views on the seriousness of the COVID-19 crisis, they also disagreed on how they saw the economy performing. Conservative economists and Republican politicians saw what they called signs of economic improvement, and with the news of progress on vaccine development that emerged in November, they felt a much smaller relief package could take the country over the hump until the COVID-19 vaccine was ready for mass distribution. Democrats disagreed, pointing out that the vaccine would not be available for most people for another six months or more, during which time thousands more people could die every day and the economy would continue to falter.

When the first COVID-19 case was reported in the United States in January, most Americans would not have predicted that by Thanksgiving over 11 million of their fellow citizens would have been infected and more than 250,000 would be dead. Neither would they have predicted that as Thanksgiving approached, a fall surge of record-breaking cases would be experienced and the virus would be running out of control. Yet, all of these things did indeed unfold. Even as the crisis was worsening at a staggering rate, Republicans and Democrats remained in stark disagreement over the threat of the virus and the steps necessary to mitigate its spread. The Congress was also at a standstill, unable to provide the needed economic relief, and the president still had not produced a national strategy for addressing the pandemic.

The partisan divide among the public also intensified dramatically as the virus spread. This surprised many political scientists and public health experts alike. They had thought that as more people became infected and the virus touched the lives of everyone, including the skeptics, the partisan gap would have begun to close. They believed that the reality of what was happening in people's families, towns, and cities would unify the nation in its fight against such a deadly threat. The hypothesis that politics would become less relevant as the pandemic crisis wore on had proven to be tragically wrong.

In mid-November, Democrats and Republicans in Congress finally agreed (sort of) that a second round of economic stimulus was needed, but they continued to disagree on what form that stimulus should take and how much it should cost. So, just as the nation's leaders had failed to develop and implement a national strategy for responding to the public health crisis, they also remained divided and disorganized when it came to addressing the economic consequences of the pandemic. In this environment, the public remained more divided and confused than ever. The United States was still running in circles and getting nowhere fast. Many hoped that the November election would bring clarity. However, like everything else in 2020, it would accentuate the confusion in a deeply divided nation as the public health disaster worsened.

COVID-19, an Election, and a Fall Spike

As the November 3 election approached, COVID dominated the news, hobbled the economy, and gripped the nation. By Election Day, it had killed more than 230,000 Americans, and it had upended everyone's daily life. Things were also getting worse by day. On Election Day, the nation recorded 91,530 new cases and 555 deaths. On November 4, the day after the election, the nation recorded 109,429 new cases for that day. The death toll had reached 233,1196. By November 13, these numbers were soaring, with the death toll topping 250,000. Over a thousand new deaths each day had become the norm. As one would expect, the pandemic was foremost on the minds of voters on Election Day.

A survey conducted by the Associated Press (AP) showed that nearly all who were surveyed said the federal government's response to the pandemic was a factor in deciding how they voted. Forty-one percent said it was the most important issue facing the country, by far the highest response to that question. Twenty-eight percent said the economy was the most important issue. However, as important as the pandemic was as an issue, opinions were divided along partisan lines just like every other issue.[43] The survey demonstrated that the people who voted for Donald Trump and the people who voted for Joe Biden did not see the same things when they considered the pandemic in relation to their voting decision (see table 6.3).

The AP survey had been conducted over several days before November 3 and had continued up until the polls closed. The data included interviews with more than 110,000 people across the United States. The results made it abundantly clear that Americans did not share the same reality when it came to COVID-19 and the country's response to it. On all questions related to the pandemic (i.e., approval of Trump's handling of the pandemic, feeling that the pandemic was under control, and support for mask requirements), Biden and Trump voters could not have disagreed more. It was as if they lived in two separate worlds. Of course, given how deeply the nation was divided along partisan lines on all issues, this was hardly surprising.

President Donald Trump hoped the predictable partisan division of the electorate would aid him in solidifying his base and diminish the impact of the pandemic on his reelection chances. He held to the view that Americans were tired of hearing about COVID. The media's focus on the spiraling death toll was, he would argue, an effort to harm him politically. He was doing a great job. He insisted, contrary to all the mounting evidence, that the United States was "rounding the corner" and the end of the public health crisis was in sight. He mocked mask wearing, made fun of his opponent for always wearing one, and flouted federal health guidelines by holding huge rallies (super-spreader events, actually) with little to no social distancing. The president's opponent, former vice president Joe Biden, took the opposite approach. He argued that Americans needed to take the virus more seriously. He discussed his plans to empower scientific experts and tackle the crisis head-on. He kept a light campaign schedule because of the pandemic. The former vice president offered a stark contrast to the Trump campaign. He made sure his events were

Table 6.3 Coronavirus and Voters in the 2020 Election

1. Is the pandemic under control?

Response	All Voters	Voted for Biden	Voted for Trump
Completely/mostly	19%	7%	91%
Somewhat under control	30%	25%	73%
Not at all under control	50%	83%	15%

2. Mask requirements?

Response	All Voters	Voted for Biden	Voted for Trump
Favor	77%	63%	36%
Oppose	23%	10%	87%

3. President Trump's handling of the pandemic?

Response	All Voters	Voted for Biden	Voted for Trump
Approve	45%	3%	96%
Disapprove	55%	90%	8%

Source: VoteCast, https://www.ap.org/en-us/topics/politics/elections/ap-votecast/about

socially distanced, and he wore a mask everywhere. Moreover, Biden repeatedly made the case that President Trump had failed to protect the country against the virus. As the candidates delivered their dueling messages, the United States suffered a new surge of infections (more than five hundred thousand over a seven-day period) just prior to Election Day. The death toll and the hospitalization rate were also on the rise.

Because of the pandemic, the simple acts of voting and counting the votes were significantly impacted. To slow the spread of the coronavirus, a record number of voters cast their votes early or by mail. Mail-in voting in particular caused some concern, as the states had differing rules on when the votes could be counted (i.e., before, during, or after the in-person vote on November 3). There were soon absurd conspiracy theories being bandied about how mail-in voting was part of a sinister effort to rig the election in favor of Joe Biden. Many of these conspiracy theories were promulgated by the president himself, and they were meant to cast doubt on the legitimacy of mail-in votes. The president understood that Democrats were expected to vote by mail in larger numbers due to their greater level of concern about the pandemic and thus the safety of in-person voting at the polls. As such, the president's strategy was to do everything he could to delegitimize or not count mail-in votes. He urged his supporters to vote on Election Day at their traditional polling places. As same-day votes were counted on November 3, the president knew he would be ahead in votes by the end of the evening. But he also knew that as the mail-in and absentee votes were counted later, he would likely fall behind. Discrediting the mail-in and absentee votes and exposing his own supporters to coronavirus risks as they voted in person seemed like a winning strategy to the president, one might suppose. Of course, as his handling of the pandemic had already made clear to both his opponents and to a majority of citizens, he was not exactly a strategic thinker so much as a narcissistic bull in a china shop.

The results of the election were slow in being finalized due to the complexity of the counting, the closeness of some of the important swing states that would decide the presidential race, and the reluctance of the media to make quick calls. It would take until Saturday, November 7, for Joe Biden to be projected as the winner and president-elect. In reality, it was not really that close in the end. Biden won 51.10 percent of the popular vote nationwide, and Trump won 47.18. The Electoral College went to Biden 306–232. More Americans voted in the 2020 presidential election than ever before (over 160 million), and the turnout percentage, while not a record, was the highest for a presidential election since 1900. The highest voter turnout in U.S. history was in 1876, when 82.6 percent of eligible voters cast ballots in the race between Republican Rutherford Hayes and Democrat Samuel Tilden. President-elect Biden received a record-setting 81 million votes, but President Trump also received a record-setting 74 million votes.

All around the country in the days following the election, Trump's lawyers and loyalists made baseless claims and allegations of systemic voter fraud and brought multiple legal challenges to the vote count, which were universally rejected in the courts. This did not stop the president and his opportunistic supporters and enablers. They continued to challenge the vote count in the battleground states, and they continued to work around the clock to create doubt and anxiety about the legitimacy of the election. The returns, despite the fake fraud claims of the president, were not controversial. Joe Biden had won. However, Democrats did not enjoy the victories they had hoped for in the Senate and state legislative races, and they lost seats in the House, although they still held a slim majority.

All of this indicated that the partisan divisions in the country remained entrenched. Concerns about the nation's failure to contain the COVID-19 pandemic had not rearranged the balance of power in the U.S. Congress, though it may have been a factor in the defeat of President Trump. Nevertheless, it is worth noting that in the middle of a pandemic, the United States had managed to pull off a national election without a significant hitch. A record number of people had voted. By all objective measures, it was a fair and controversy-free election. Only the efforts of President Trump and his enablers to undermine the confidence of the nation in the result, to literally attack and undermine democracy itself, soiled the election and its aftermath.

As the postelection weeks unfolded, President Trump tirelessly promoted a fictive voter fraud narrative as he did his best to undermine the popular will of the people and the vote. That effort—and golfing—consumed all his time. The COVID-19 drama, in the meantime, was entering a new and even more dangerous phase. The time between Election Day and the January 20, 2021, inauguration of Joe Biden as president would follow a familiar pattern. As had been the case throughout 2020, the spread of the virus and the rising number of deaths would continue uninterrupted in a leadership vacuum.

Conclusion: The Worst Was Yet to Come

By the second week of November 2020, there was no denying that COVID-19 was back with a vengeance in much of the world. However, authorities and public health experts around the globe warned that the worst may be yet to come. Japan, whose daily COVID-19 infections had numbered in the low hundreds only weeks before, had seen a marked uptick in cases. On Friday, November 13, it had hit a new daily high (1,693) for the second straight day. South Korea and Indonesia were also setting new records, and Europe was showing an alarming upward trend in infections. Daily records for new infections were being set in Russia (21,983), Great Britain (33,470), Italy (30,000), and Greece (3,000). On November 12, the United States set a new high for the third straight day with 153,496 infections. More than a dozen states had doubled their caseloads over the previous two weeks.

News reports in early November included promising reports that an effective vaccine was closer to fruition. Pfizer's and Moderna's disclosures of successful early data from large-scale clinical trials of their COVID-19 vaccines sent the stock markets soaring. But that did not negate the fact that as winter descended on some regions, the pandemic would worsen, as people were more likely to gather indoors and spend more time in warmer, less ventilated areas, allowing the coronavirus to spread more easily. With access to a vaccine still some months away, experts stressed that measures to contain infections must remain in place. The country's top infectious disease specialist, Dr Anthony Fauci, concurred with this assessment: "Now we need to double down on the public health measures as we're waiting for the vaccine."[44]

By Friday, November 27, more than 13 million people had been infected in the United States since the pandemic began, and nearly 267,000 had died. On that day, over 200,000 new cases were recorded, another new single-day record for the United States. Most experts were saying that the number of people infected was likely far higher, as many asymptomatic individuals never get reflected in the official counts. Many also feared that the daily death toll would soon hit 3,000 per day. That would be the equivalent of a September 11 attack every single day. Despite warnings not to travel over the Thanksgiving holiday, millions of Americans did so anyway. As a result, medical personnel braced for what they feared would be a new spurt of infections in the weeks between Thanksgiving and Christmas. Dr. Anthony Fauci warned that "we may see a surge upon a surge." On a popular Sunday morning network news program, he said, "We don't want to frighten people, but that's just the reality. We said that these things would happen as we got into the cold weather and as we began traveling, and they've happened."[45] Such a surge would follow the pattern of spikes in infections after the Memorial Day and Fourth of July holidays.

As the fall wave was intensifying and cases surged, hospitals were already at or near capacity. The nation's most valuable resources in fighting the pandemic, health care professionals, were being stretched to their limit. Public officials and public health experts expressed a growing frustration at the continued unwillingness of too many Americans to follow guidance aimed at curbing the virus's spread.

In the midst of all that was happening in the aftermath of the election, and as the United States plunged deeper into the worst public health crisis it had faced in over one hundred years, President Trump refused to take charge. He showed no interest in and made no effort to engage in any efforts to address what appeared to be an out-of-control public health emergency. His time was spent on a fruitless effort to win an election he had already convincingly lost. President Trump, his family, his advisers, and his various enablers spent all their time and energy desperately trying to overturn the results of a free and fair election. He was not at all interested in actually doing the job of president, especially where the pandemic was concerned. By all appearances, he was missing in action when it came to addressing the postelection surge in cases. It was, to put it bluntly, an especially staggering and surreal failure of leadership given the new surge in cases. But that was consistent with his performance throughout the public health crisis and the subsequent economic turmoil that accompanied it. Even for a president who had downplayed and lied about the true nature of the pandemic and repeatedly predicted the virus would just go away, this failure to lead and act was unprecedented and inexcusable. His absence without leave from his responsibilities became more inexcusable by the day as the pandemic raged across the country and the nation was breaking every record for new cases, deaths, and hospitalizations.

As December arrived, Americans were facing strict new coronavirus restrictions all around the country. Public health officials were bracing for a disastrous worsening of the nationwide surge because of holiday travel and gatherings over the Thanksgiving weekend. They had pleaded with Americans to stay home over the holiday and not to gather with anyone who did not live with them. Nevertheless, more people traveled than at any time during the pandemic. On the Sunday after Thanksgiving, some 1.2 million people passed through the nation's airports. Others who had taken to the highways to gather with family and friends were also returning home. Expecting the worst, public health officials urged all these travelers (and the persons they had visited) to get tested over the week ahead as a precaution. At least 90,000 people in the United States were already in the nation's hospitals with the virus by the Sunday after Thanksgiving. Hospitals and health care professionals were pushed to their limit. The weeks ahead looked as if they might be the darkest weeks of the pandemic. The U.S. response to COVID-19 was on target to completely derail unless the nation could apply the brakes with all of its collective might. The persistent failure of the United States throughout 2020 to control the spread of the virus was about to reach its inevitable climax.

CHAPTER SEVEN

The Darkest Days

For too long, humanity has acted with an outrageous lack of responsibility. We wanted everything for ourselves: greed really. We failed to look at the overall picture and did not take into consideration those with whom we share the world.

—Sheri Arison, Israeli businesswoman and philanthropist

If you're going through hell, keep going.

—Winston Churchill

Introduction

December brought a number of somber milestones in the United States' ongoing and frustrating battle to control the COVID-19 pandemic. By December 22, the United States had seen cases surpass the 18-million mark. There had been a total of 18,134,027 COVID-19 recorded cases as of that Tuesday morning, according to data provided by Johns Hopkins University, and the death toll had risen to 321,301. Hospitalizations on that day had jumped by 1,750 to a record of 115,351. The daily count of new cases had reached a high of 280,514 on December 11, and the highest death toll for a single day, 3,611, had occurred on December 16. Simply put, things were not good. But everything that was happening was very predictable. The scientific experts had told us back in October that COVID-19 could kill 3,000 Americans a day in December. They had also warned that there would be a worsening of the nationwide surge in cases and deaths because of holiday travel and gatherings over the Thanksgiving weekend. But even in this darkest hour, some good news did emerge.

Two vaccine candidates that were said to be effective against coronavirus were approved by the Federal Drug Administration. The first to be approved came from the U.S. pharmaceutical giant Pfizer, which reported that its vaccine had demonstrated 95 percent effectiveness in clinical trials. The second to be approved was from Moderna, another U.S. drug developer, which reported that its vaccine was 94 percent effective. Both companies had tested an initial dose plus a subsequent booster dose several weeks later, with few if any serious side effects reported. Pfizer expected to produce up to 50 million vaccine doses in December 2020 and 1.3 billion in 2021. Moderna planned to ship 20 million doses in December 2020 and another 500 million to 1 billion in 2021.

As this news broke, and was understandably celebrated, people needed to be reminded that this was just the first leg of a long journey still ahead. Convincing people to take the vaccines would be the next step in that journey. Sixty-three percent of U.S. adults expressed safety concerns over a coronavirus vaccine, according to a Harris Poll survey from October 19, with 40 percent of respondents specifically worrying that development had been too fast.[1] Some people were reportedly concerned about possible side effects. Life would not begin to return to normal until enough people had received the vaccine. Scientists noted that herd immunity, meaning that at least 60 percent to 70 percent of the population is immune, could only be achieved if enough people were vaccinated. So long as enough people took the vaccine to reach that level, it would not matter whether a few people objected or declined to take the vaccine.

Assuming that people were eager to be vaccinated, the logistics of getting that done were complex enough to mean that it could be the summer or fall of 2021 before significant numbers of people were vaccinated. This would make it necessary to continue masking and maintaining social distancing protocols. Even with the light at the end of tunnel provided by the vaccines, things would still get much worse in the short term. The United States was averaging nearly three thousand deaths per day as the vaccines became available. Tens of thousands more lives would be lost in the months to come, and the vaccines would not be able to stop that. The country would need to remain vigilant. It would still need a national plan and national leadership to manage the challenges, especially with respect to vaccine distribution, in the months ahead. It had not had these things throughout 2020, and the United States had paid a dear price for that and would continue to do so.

By December 19, new concerns occupied the minds of scientists and hinted at unwelcomed twists in the road ahead. The coronavirus had mutated. This is actually a natural and expected development. Viruses always mutate, or develop small changes, as they reproduce and move through a population. Most mutations are trivial. They amount to a change of one or two letters in the genetic alphabet that do not make significant differences in the ability of the virus to cause disease. But worry had been growing since December 19. It was on that day that British Prime Minister Boris Johnson warned of a new coronavirus strain that was spreading through England. This strain, or variant, was said to be spreading more easily than earlier ones, and it was becoming the dominant one because it was outcompeting the other strains, moving faster, and infecting more people. First reports said there was no increase in the severity of COVID-19 from this new strain, and there was no reason to doubt that treatments and the new vaccines would be effective against it. But it would be important to be alert to the possibility of any changes along these lines. The greatest concern is that when a virus mutates by changing the proteins on its surface to help it escape from drugs or the immune system, it may become very different from previous versions. It may become more severe or perhaps less. In this case, the initial assessment was that this mutation had given the new variant the advantage of spreading more easily. In response, dozens of countries barred flights from the United Kingdom (the United States did not), and Southern England was placed under strict lockdown measures. The first case of the new strain in the United States was confirmed in Colorado on December 29.

The Centers for Disease Control and Prevention (CDC) urged Americans to avoid traveling over the Christmas holidays to prevent another nationwide surge in coronavirus cases, but many insisted on coming or going. Cases were rising, hospitalizations were increasing, and deaths were mounting. Americans were told by the experts of the urgent need to try to bend the curve to stop these exponential increases. But an estimated 85 million Americans traveled over the holidays anyway. This would, of course, lead to an unmanageable spike in cases by mid-January and well into February. By December 28, the United States had topped 19 million cases. This represented a 1.1 million increase in cases in just the previous six days. In that same six days, the death toll had climbed by over 15,000 to 336,761. The post-Christmas surge that was inevitable, given the holiday travel, would see these numbers explode. To the very end, the misery of 2020 would continue unabated. Was there any reason to expect that 2021 would be any better?

Finally, a Plan to Combat COVID?

Joseph R. Biden was elected the forty-sixth president of the United States on November 3, 2020. Biden had served thirty-six years in the U.S.

Senate and eight years as vice president. During the Obama administration, the vice president had been a part of the U.S. H1N1 pandemic response. He was well versed on the Obama administration's pandemic planning and the pandemic playbook that had been produced in that ongoing effort. He was also acutely aware of the failures of the Trump administration in its response to the COVID-19 pandemic. Most importantly, the president-elect had a sense of urgency about developing something that should have been a first priority of the failed Trump administration. He knew that a national plan of action, driven by science, was desperately needed.

The president-elect laid out a three-point plan to begin defeating the coronavirus pandemic during his first one hundred days in office. First, he committed to signing an executive order the day he was sworn in to require Americans to wear masks on buses and trains crossing state lines as well as in federal buildings. But he wavered on imposing a national face mask requirement, suggesting that this was beyond the authority of the federal government to do. Second, he pledged to distribute at least one hundred million COVID vaccine shots during the first one hundred days of his presidency. After the vaccines were first given to health workers and people who live and work in long-term care facilities, he emphasized that he would prioritize educators. This related to the third goal, which was to enable "the majority of our schools" to reopen within that time and to remain open. He also called on Congress to devote the funding needed to make it safe for students and teachers to return to classrooms.[2]

The president-elect also emphasized the need for the federal government to work with the states in a more coordinated effort to manage things. He spoke of working with the fifty state governors to provide federal guidance and to enlist their support for state mask mandates and other measures that were needed to stem the spread of the virus. Unlike President Trump, Biden emphasized that a mask was the most potent weapon against the virus; he also emphasized the importance of following the science in every step taken in response to the pandemic. As far as Biden was concerned, the debate over face masks highlighted the importance of listening to science. He knew that public health officials had concluded that defiance of the advice to wear masks was the major reason the rate of infection in the United States far exceeded that of most other nations.

Resistance to mask wearing and mask mandates had begun to wane among state and local elected officials, but some Republican governors were still reluctant to implement statewide mandates. These governors had followed President Trump in "playing down" the pandemic. As previously discussed, President Trump had often ignored the advice of his

COVID-19 task force. He often contradicted his administration's public health experts, and he even mocked mask wearing. Public health leaders had grown increasingly weary with the Trump administration's hostility to scientific advice. This had made it impossible to control the pandemic. They now welcomed the new tone from the president-elect. They also welcomed the new COVID-19 advisory board Biden announced shortly after the November election.[3] These appointments stressed the need to bring much-needed competence to the federal government's pandemic response.

The president-elect appointed an advisory board of top public health experts to guide his transition team's COVID-19 planning. The advisory board would be led by three prominent longtime Biden advisers: former Food and Drug Administration commissioner David Kessler, former surgeon general Vivek Murthy, and Marcella Nunez-Smith, an associate professor of internal medicine, public health, and management at Yale University. Kessler and Murthy would serve as cochairs of the twelve-member task force. Also appointed to the task force was Rick Bright, an immunologist who directed the Biomedical Advanced Research and Development Authority. He had been fired by the Trump administration when he went public with criticisms that the administration had not taken the pandemic and the science surrounding it seriously, and he had accused officials of ignoring warnings about the pandemic.[4] In addition to guiding the Biden administration's response to the pandemic, the new board would address a need that had been ignored throughout all of 2020. It would consult and work with state and local officials to gauge the public health steps needed to bring the virus under control. Another highly respected expert, and the nation's top infectious disease expert, Dr. Anthony Fauci, was also invited to join the new Biden administration as its chief medical adviser. Biden noted that he had "asked him to stay on in the exact same role as he's had for the past several presidents," and "I asked him to be a chief medical adviser for me as well and be part of the COVID-19 team."[5]

As previously mentioned, Dr. Fauci, along with another highly praised expert, Dr. Deborah Birx, served on the Trump administration's COVID-19 task force. Together, they were the leading voices of science charged with guiding that body. Fauci had often pushed back against President Trump's misstatements throughout the year. True to the science, this won him even more respect from peers and the public. Birx, on the other hand, seemed to think it was necessary to maintain her job and influence by not publicly contradicting Trump's misstatements and policies while attempting to ensure that the public still got quality information. Her failure to effectively push back on President Trump's wild misinformation bursts severely undercut her credibility with the medical and public health communities. Dr Birx was interested in working within the new administration to address the pandemic, but her perceived failure to push back against President Trump's misinformation throughout the year of crisis left Biden and many in his planning circle wary of welcoming her to the team. Her credibility was seen as severely compromised.

Members of the new task force, along with scientists and public health experts generally, felt that in addition to battling the pandemic, another of President-elect Biden's major challenges would be rebuilding public trust in federal health agencies, such as the Food and Drug Administration (FDA) and the CDC. Public health agencies had been subject to intense political meddling and control under Trump. In fact, the president seemed to go out of his way to discredit the scientific expertise of these agencies and to control their public pronouncements to suit his political purposes and interests. The CDC, for example, had long been viewed as one of the world's premier health agencies. But its reputation had taken a jarring hit during the pandemic as its guidance became politicized by the president's political appointees. President Trump himself undercut CDC Director Robert Redfield on the importance of mask use, and the department's top scientists were all but sidelined and silenced as the COVID-19 pandemic ravaged the country. To make matters worse, the outgoing U.S. president was working to sabotage his successor.

President Trump was in denial about his election defeat. His lies about nonexistent mass coordinated election fraud, the more than sixty lawsuits challenging the vote count in key swing states (all of which failed for lack of evidence), and his ongoing and corrupt efforts to undermine democracy culminated in his strangling of the rituals of transferring power between administrations. For weeks after the election and his refusal to concede, President Trump's appointee at the head of the General Services Administration (GSA) would not recognize Biden as the president-elect and would not allow the transition to proceed, as would be a matter of routine under normal circumstances. In the last week of November, the GSA, under growing public pressure, finally allowed the transition process to begin. President Trump assented and authorized the federal government to initiate the Biden transition. But he did not concede defeat, as he was determined to carry on with his reality-challenged but diligent effort. The president was intent on constructing a stolen election myth. While this might not enable him to overturn the results, as he hoped, it would at least allow him to retain his pride and build a rationale for his running again in 2024. Even as the transition formally began, almost a month late, the degree of cooperation from the Trump administration with the Biden transition team was inconsistent at best.[6,7]

President Trump's postelection behavior and conspiracy theories were not just the democracy-damaging aberrations of a madman; they also had a practical fallout. There was growing concern that these efforts to overturn the election results would complicate and negatively impact the transition. They might also, it was feared, complicate and hinder the Biden pandemic planning process. Some feared that this could slow the delivery of the vaccines when they became available.[8] The vaccine operation would be massively complex and difficult, and the effort would require a high level of public trust. Public health officials rightly worried that the Trumpian efforts to sabotage the transition would handicap the incoming administration in its efforts to manage the pandemic and perhaps also get a lot of people killed. While President Trump was working to hold on to the White House, even if it meant weakening democratic institutions and wreaking deadly havoc on the nation, it is equally important and concerning to note what he was not doing as December saw the pandemic entering its darkest hours.

During each presidential transition period, Americans are reminded that we have only one president at a time. But during the 2020 transition period, it appeared that the United States had no president at all. Since Election Day, Donald Trump had done virtually nothing. His official schedule on most days had been empty. There were no signs of presidential activity, no public statements, and no substantive activity. There was a constant flow of baseless conspiracy theories about a rigged election on Twitter, and there had been a vigorous flurry of golfing. Golf and a nonstop barrage of tweeting and retweeting about disproven election conspiracy theories were all one heard of Donald Trump from November 4 to January 20 and the inauguration of Joe Biden. With a massive pandemic entering its deadliest, costliest, and most debilitating phase, President Trump would remain largely silent about the December surge in coronavirus infections, hospitalizations, and deaths.

As the White House proceeded with plans to host numerous indoor holiday receptions and parties (just as public health authorities urged ordinary Americans to avoid or limit holiday gatherings), President Trump and his administration made no visible efforts to address the worsening crisis, although White House Press Secretary Kayleigh McEnany did take the time to criticize new lockdown measures being reimplemented in some parts of the country. President Trump did briefly emerge from his golf and Twitter addictions to claim personal credit for the Pfizer and Moderna vaccines when they were announced, but he could not be bothered to make any visible efforts to curb the surge in virus cases. He would mostly stick to his schedule of golfing, tweeting insane conspiracy theories, making unfounded claims about election rigging, and working with an assortment of his enablers to overturn the will of the people as expressed in the November vote. All in all, it was not the most inspiring example of presidential leadership during a national crisis.[9]

President Donald Trump was publicly disengaged from the battle against coronavirus at the exact moment when the disease was tearing across the country at its most alarming rate yet. His silence during the spike in cases as well as his refusal to coordinate with the Biden transition team on pandemic issues were points of concern to the experts and public alike. Even with the good news represented by the vaccine approvals, many worried that the results of their rollout could be diminished by a lack of coordination between the outgoing and the incoming administrations. To many, especially President Trump's most ardent critics, it seemed that a president who had downplayed the danger of this pandemic from its very beginning was now, on his temper-tantrum-fueled way out the door, determined to leave death and destruction in his wake. Whatever his intentions, there was ample reason to fear such an outcome. The December surge had taken the danger to a new and very threatening level.

Surge upon Surge: What "Bad" Really Looked Like

As vaccines began to be slowly distributed across the nation, the level of new COVID-19 cases in the United States had hit a plateau over the two-week Christmas holiday break. Experts also warned that the country should expect another surge in mid-January due to holiday gatherings as well as the number of people who traveled during the break. By the first week of the new year, the United States had confirmed more than 21 million COVID-19 cases since the pandemic began. U.S. COVID-19–related deaths now exceeded 356,000. That included the 2,048 deaths recorded on January 4. The month of December had seen more than 78,000 COVID-related deaths. This was the highest monthly total since the pandemic began.[10] The previous week alone had seen 1.5 million new COVID-19 cases and more than 18,000 deaths. The Institute for Health Metrics and Evaluation (IHME) predicted the United States would top 560,000 deaths by April 1 if the current conditions were to continue.[11] As bad as these numbers were, public health experts warned of another massive surge in cases as the Christmas and New Year's holidays faded into the rearview mirror. Holiday travel and gatherings would surely amplify the crisis. It seemed that Americans just could not resist putting themselves at more and more risk of being infected with the coronavirus. The experiences of states across the country in December signaled that there would be some dark days ahead.

California, the most populous state in the country, also became one of the nation's worst epicenters for the disease in December. It was setting new records for cases, hospitalizations, and deaths almost every day. Things were so bad in Southern California that some patients were being treated in hospital tents, and doctors had begun discussing the need to begin rationing care. Hospitals were running out of room, intensive care units were filled to capacity, and health care workers were overwhelmed; by January, it had become impossible for some of them to admit every new arriving patient or to treat every case. California, like most states, had begun providing its initial vaccine allotments to health care workers, but immunizations were not expected to have a dramatic impact on infection spread for months, after broader distribution took place.[12]

Alabama recorded almost a third of its 2020 coronavirus cases in the month of December. Over 109,000 of its 361,226 confirmed and probable COVID-19 cases were reported in December. The December surge came after the Thanksgiving holiday, and health officials were concerned that caseloads would continue to grow in January from the fallout of Christmas and New Year's travel and gatherings. The number of people in Alabama hospitals rose from 1,731 on November 30 to a record 2,813 on December 30. Over 47 percent of beds in state intensive care units were occupied by COVID-19 patients.[13]

Through the first two weeks of December, Tennessee had posted a seven-day average of 7,978 new cases per day, a 68 percent increase. Tennessee was also home to nine of the twenty metro areas across the country that were, when adjusted for population size, seeing the fastest-growing outbreaks in the United States. Despite an alarming surge in cases, Tennessee's Republican governor, Bill Lee, continued to rebuff advice from local, state, and federal health advisers on the issuing of a statewide mask mandate.[14]

Across the nation, New Year's Day brought news of a crush of COVID-19 patients that were pushing hospitals beyond their limits. In Los Angeles, there were reports of doctors treating patients on oxygen in waiting rooms after running out of beds. From Texas came the news of patients who needed to be transferred from small facilities to larger metropolitan hospitals. But the lack of hospital space saw patients having to sit in limbo for hours or days before being transferred, putting them at risk of developing complications from delays. Desperate smaller hospitals had begun to fly patients as far as Albuquerque, New Mexico, and Oklahoma City for an open bed. From North Carolina, one heard about the rising number of intensive care patients in Charlotte that had forced doctors to save ICU beds for the "sickest of the sickest" from COVID and find somewhere else in hospitals for all other critically ill patients. In short, the surge of coronavirus cases across the nation was crowding large metro hospitals with COVID-19 patients, pushing occupancy against the limits of space, and overwhelming nurses and doctors. Up to 60 percent of ICU patients in some metro areas were critically ill from COVID-19.[15] Many hospitals had reached the crisis point and were having to make tough decisions about patient care. To make matters worse, the coming weeks were expected to further stress hospitals and health care providers as another postholiday surge (on top of an already difficult to manage surge) would be inevitable as the months of January and February wore on.

During a December 29 interview on CNN, Dr. Anthony Fauci expressed the worry that COVID-19 case numbers had gotten too high during the December surge. "We're in such a surge that has just gotten out of control in many respects," he explained. "If you look at the history . . . we had a surge in the late winter, early spring, another surge in the early summer. We're, right now, in a surge whose incline, whose inflection, is very sharp." Fauci, noting that the ongoing surge had created an incredibly "difficult situation," worried that things were about to get worse.[16] "The reason I'm concerned, and my colleagues in public health are concerned also, is that we very well might see a post-seasonal—in the sense of Christmas/New Year's–surge." This would, Fauci feared, bring a surge upon a surge in the weeks to come.[17] As 2020 came to an end, and even with the positive news about a vaccine rollout, a perfect storm seemed to have created the conditions necessary for a very troubling beginning to the new year. For that matter, the vaccine rollout did not seem to be going very smoothly either.

Operation Warp Speed, the federal government's plan (a public-private partnership) for vaccine production and distribution, was not quite working as had been hoped. Warp Speed had reached the goal of actually having a vaccine to distribute in an impressively short time, thanks to the scientists and companies working to develop it. But it was soon apparent that the nation was struggling with the critical step of getting the vaccine into people's arms. Operation Warp Speed had the ambitious goal of immunizing 20 million people by the end of December. By the first week of January, about 15 million vaccine doses had been distributed to the states, but only a little over 4.5 million people had received their first dose. Snafus were first observed when states received smaller shipments than they had expected. Pfizer immediately put out a press release saying that the issue was not that doses were not available to ship: "We have millions more doses sitting in our warehouse but, as of now, we have not received any shipment instructions for additional doses." A few days later, Operation Warp Speed's chief operating officer, Gustave Perna, explained that the issue was "a delay between what is available and what is releasable." Apparently, he had failed to account for the fact that the FDA needed to receive a quality control analysis before each lot of shipments went out.[18]

But this was only the beginning of the glitches that would complicate the vaccine rollout. Even where doses were available, they were not being effectively allocated. Breakdowns in the process of booking appointments, confusion about the process, a shortage of staff to administer the doses, too few centers for vaccine distribution, and a lack of federal guidance that led to inadequate planning at the state and local levels were among the things that contributed to what could only be described as an embarrassing failure to get the vaccine into arms.[19] At the rate things were going, it would take almost ten years to inoculate enough Americans to get the pandemic under control.

President-elect Joe Biden criticized the Trump administration for falling short in providing the necessary leadership to expedite the vaccination process. "We are grateful to the companies, doctors, scientists, researchers and clinical trial participants and Operation Warp Speed for developing the vaccines quickly," he said. "But as I long feared and warned, the effort to distribute and administer the vaccine is not progressing as it should." President Trump tweeted in reply that it was "up to the States to distribute the vaccines," and, for good measure, he repeated the false claim that Biden had "failed with the Swine Flu" during the Obama administration.[20] A tweet evading responsibility and a lie were the extent of the sitting president's response to the growing concerns about vaccine distribution.

If the goal was to vaccinate as many people as possible in a systematic and equitable way, then the December rollout of the vaccines was a failure. The states, working through their local public health departments and hospitals, were simply ill-equipped and underresourced to handle the vaccination effort. Many observers, noting the lack of and absolute need for planning, coordination, and execution, suggested that it was time to call out the troops. The National Guard is called on in times of natural disasters. It was suggested by many that their expertise may be of help in planning, coordinating, and executing the efficient distribution and administering of vaccinations. It was time to use school buildings, parking lots, and convention centers to serve as vaccine hubs. It was also time to recognize the impracticality of relying on the overburdened heath care system to manage this type of massive effort. It was already at its breaking point dealing with the treatment of patients. Clearly, any such efforts to improve the situation would have to wait for January 20 and the beginning of the Biden administration.

In addition to the December spikes in infections, hospitalizations, and deaths; the expected postholiday spikes; and the failure to get the approved vaccines into the arms of citizens, there was another cause for concern as one year ended and a new one began: the virus had mutated. By December 2020, a new strain of the coronavirus that causes COVID-19 was reported in the news media. The particular strain that was reported at that time was first detected in southeastern England in September 2020. By December, it had become the most common version of the coronavirus in England, accounting for about 60 percent of new COVID-19 cases. This new strain also appeared in Denmark, the Netherlands, and other European countries, and a similar variant emerged in South Africa.[21] The new strain, or the mutated virus, seemed to spread faster from person to person, but it did not appear any more likely to cause severe disease or death. There was some concern that experts in areas where the new strain was appearing had found an increased number of cases in children. There was, they cautioned, no need to fear this variant had a special propensity to infect or cause disease in children, but everything amounted to mere speculation at that point in time. We would need to be vigilant in monitoring such shifts.[22]

By the first week of January, the new strain had contributed to push Europe to a new tipping point in the course of the pandemic. The coronavirus was spreading very fast across the continent, and the arrival of a new variant had contributed greatly to an alarming spike in the number of cases.[23] By the end of December, the new and more transmissible strain of the coronavirus had been identified in several U.S. states. On December 29, Colorado was the first state to report a case of the new COVID-19 variant. Colorado was followed by California on December 30, Florida on December 31, New York on January 4, and Georgia on January 5. Because there was no travel history associated with these first cases of the new strain, it was believed that these were not isolated cases. The new strain, it was thought, had arrived in the United States, and it would no doubt be only a matter of time before it was prevalent. This new variant, known as the B.1.1.7 strain, had been detected in at least thirty-three countries by the beginning of the new year. Cases had been confirmed in Australia, Belgium, Brazil, Canada, Chile, China, Denmark, Finland, France, Germany, Iceland, India, Ireland, Israel, Italy, Japan, Jordan, Lebanon, Malta, the Netherlands, Norway, Pakistan, Portugal, Singapore, South Korea, Spain, Sweden, Switzerland, Taiwan, Turkey, the United Arab Emirates, the United Kingdom, and the United States.[24] As this news was circulating, the CDC in the United States was not yet confirming that the new strain was anything more than a few travel-related cases as opposed to community spread.

The CDC had warned that the U.K. variant might already be spreading within the United States because there was still ongoing travel between the United States and nations where it was prevalent. Should the new variant become widespread in the United States, as it surely would, this would be a matter of great concern. Why? Though there was no evidence to date that the new strain caused a more intense illness or led to a higher fatality rate, faster transmission would mean more cases, which would lead to higher hospitalization rates and more deaths.[25] Given the December surge, the expected postholiday surge, the failures associated with the vaccine rollout, and the fact that hospitals were already being pushed past their limits, this could only make a bad situation worse. No less an expert than Dr. Anthony Fauci had declared that the COVID pandemic was already out of control in the United States.

How out of control was the pandemic at the beginning of 2021? For months, the United States had been the country with the highest COVID-19 case count and death toll. As of January 14, 2021, 384,794 American fatalities had been reported out of 23,079,163 cases. Cases had peaked at around 75,000 per day in July, dropping in the fall before once again spiking upward. On January 13 alone, 229,610 new COVID cases were confirmed. Hospitalizations had also skyrocketed to 130,383. January 13 also saw 4,022 fatalities, making it the third day in a row that the daily death toll had topped 4,000. The highest daily total had been 4,500 on January 12. Since the beginning of the new year, in just the first couple of weeks of 2021, about 40,000 Americans had died of COVID-19, and over 200,000 new cases were being added nationwide each day. As these numbers were sinking in, the CDC was projecting that the American death toll could reach 477,000 by the end of the first week in February.[26] These numbers made it clear that the COVID pandemic was indeed out of control. But, as December became January, it was not the only thing out of control in the United States.

Political Mayhem

On January 14, the United Press International (UPI) reported that the previous week had seen another million workers in the United States file new unemployment claims. According to the U.S. Labor Department, that was the largest weekly number of claims since August 2020. It will be recalled from our discussion in the previous chapter that the CARES

Act, passed by the Congress in March 2020, provided $2 trillion of federal economic stimulus to help offset the economic fallout from the pandemic. It would soon become apparent that more help was needed. The Democrat House had passed a $3 trillion package, called the HEROES Act, in May. In the Senate, as we noted, this was a nonstarter. Republicans in the Senate objected to the price tag and, in addition, felt that the economy would recover by the fall. They also objected to providing federal funding for state and local governments to assist them in maintaining essential services. With budget deadlines for the new fiscal year rapidly approaching, many states faced unanticipated shortfalls as a result of the crisis. Months of impasse followed. Negotiations between the House and the Senate came down to the wire as twelve million people were set to lose unemployment benefits the day after Christmas. With time running out, lawmakers reached a last-minute compromise. They agreed to a $900 billion package that included another round of stimulus checks ($600) for Americans who had earned up to $75,000 in 2019 and some badly needed jobless benefits for struggling Americans. A part of the relief package also included an extension on the eviction moratorium. This measure would no doubt help Americans in the near term, but it stopped far short of mitigating the economic fallout that households would continue to endure during the pandemic.

The narrowness of the limited $900 billion compromise package that emerged meant that President-elect Joe Biden's administration would have to immediately deal with providing a more substantial relief package. This would, of necessity, include dealing with the long-delayed priority of supporting state and local governments. Critics of the package also said the bill did not go far enough in providing direct aid to those most impacted by the economic downturn. They regarded the compromise as a limited first step, not a final solution, for the much larger and still growing problem. It was, they suggested, a bridge to get the nation to a Biden presidency, where something that was far more intense and larger in scale could be done.

The inability of Republicans and Democrats in the Congress to agree on the need for or the size of a COVID-19 economic relief package was not at all unexpected. The legislative process had long ago broken down and come to a grinding halt. This had long been situation normal in the Congress. Expecting compromise and significant legislative action addressing the nation's most acute problems had long been something that bordered on fantasy. Partisan trenches were dug so deep that neither side could see, much less talk to, the other. As bad as a broken legislative system might be during a crisis, a much worse political tragedy was unfolding that would tear at the very fabric of the republic.

President Trump had said little (i.e., nothing) about the pandemic or the December spikes in infections, hospitalizations, and deaths since the first Tuesday in November. But he spoke, tweeted, and speechified without taking so much as a breath for the two months after the November 3 election. He lost that election. It was, by all objective measures and official assessments, a free and fair election. But Donald Trump refused to accept that reality. "I won the election!" the president tweeted just before midnight on the Sunday night after the election. In the days and weeks to follow, President Trump repeatedly attacked the validity of the election results, tweeting that this was a "rigged election," a "Rigged and Corrupt Election," and a "Rigged Election Hoax." He also tweeted that this was the "most fraudulent Election in history" and that the results are "fake."[27]

The president would persist in his great election lie for the next two months. He declared to all who would listen that the election was stolen by corrupt Democrats. This was the "big lie." To support this big lie, numerous little lies were told noisily and repeatedly. To hear Trump and his allies tell it, the election was "rigged," the voting machines were "fixed," and "dead people were voting." As the president told it, he had won the election in a landslide. None of these statements—absolutely none of them—were supported by a shred of evidence.

Lie after lie and fiction after fiction was tweeted daily. The president wildly tweeted that there are "millions of ballots that have been altered by Democrats, only for Democrats." There was zero evidence of any ballot altering. He tweeted that "All of the mechanical 'glitches' that took place on Election Night were really them getting caught trying to steal votes." There was no evidence of anyone trying to use voting technology to steal votes. Statements by Trump administration officials and state election officials concluded that "there is no evidence that any voting system deleted or lost votes, changed votes, or was in any way compromised." He tweeted about absentee ballot fraud in Philadelphia. Officials found no evidence of a fraud scheme in Philadelphia. The president would claim that the election was "stolen" in part by a voting equipment and software company, Dominion Voting Systems, which he suggested was biased against him and that also has "bum equipment." Again, there was no evidence of any wrongdoing by Dominion and no evidence that any issues with Dominion's technology affected vote counts. The recount of the vote in Georgia was called a "fake recount." The endless number of false claims made by the president were all easily disproven.[28]

In addition to his tweets and public proclamations of victory, the president filed an endless stream of lawsuits seeking judicial rulings in his favor that would, if not overturn the election, give legitimacy to his claims.

The vast majority of the lawsuits were in six pivotal battleground states that Biden won: Arizona, Georgia, Michigan, Nevada, Pennsylvania, and Wisconsin. These lawsuits were dismissed for several reasons. A few were dismissed for lack of standing, and most were dismissed for a complete lack of any evidence based on the merits of the voter fraud allegations. The decisions were rendered by Democratic-appointed and Republican-appointed judges alike—including federal judges and Supreme Court justices appointed by Donald Trump.[29] Despite all the lawsuits, the two months of false allegations about a "rigged" election, and the president's refusal to concede the election and recognize Joe Biden as the president-elect, the Electoral College vote remained 306 for Biden and 232 for Trump. Joe Biden had won eighty-one million popular votes to Donald Trump's seventy-four million popular votes.

The U.S. Department of Homeland Security's Cybersecurity and Infrastructure Security Agency had declared from the beginning that the 2020 election had been the most secure in American history. It was concluded that there was no evidence of widespread voter fraud or irregularities. Still, the president persisted. The man who said he had "played down" the pandemic because he did not want to cause panic was hell-bent on causing as much panic as he could about the election. Despite the conclusion of every reliable source, including federal and state courts, state and local election officials (including every Republican election official), and federal Cybersecurity and Infrastructure Security officials that the election had been fair and free of any significant irregularities, Mr. Trump persisted. The "big lie" he promoted was, sadly, believed by many citizens, especially by Trump supporters. In fact, in a January 15 Pew Research Center survey, a large majority of those who voted for Donald Trump incorrectly believed their candidate had received the most votes cast by eligible voters in enough states to win the election. There was no subgroup of Trump voters in which a majority, or even a substantial minority, accepted that Biden received the most votes cast by eligible voters in enough states to win the election. An astounding 75 percent of Trump voters said that he had definitely or probably won the election. Trump voters, persuaded by their leader's torrent of lies, believed beyond any doubt that there had been widespread voter fraud.[30]

President Trump's strategy all along had been to create panic among his followers about the election results. This strategy was in evidence well before the election itself. Seeing troubling polls, and suspecting he might be in some trouble, he had begun throughout the summer of 2020 to ratchet up his predictions of fraud in the coming November election. These predictions were made without any supporting evidence. The president harped on the notion that mail-in ballots, which would be in more wide-spread use as Americans faced limits on their movements because of the pandemic, were "a disaster for our country." He warned that mail carriers would be held up as they delivered ballots, that ballots would be counterfeited by enemies both foreign and domestic, and that the only way he could lose the election was if it was rigged. "This will be, in my opinion, the most corrupt election in the history of our country," the president repeated to cheering believers throughout the summer and fall.[31] One is left to wonder what the positive impact might have been if the president had spent as much time and energy communicating accurate information about COVID-19 and effectively communicating the advice of public health experts over the summer and fall. There is no wondering about the impact of the president's "big lie" about election fraud. That would be made manifestly clear on January 6, 2021.

As President Trump saw his challenges to the election results failing in the courts of the land, his repeated efforts to twist the arms of Republican election officials failing to overturn the vote in contested states, and the inevitability of Joe Biden's inauguration becoming more and more apparent to him, he resorted to one last Hail Mary to overturn the election results. January 6 was the day that the U.S. Congress would record the Electoral College votes and formally make Joe Biden the forty-sixth president of the United States. This is primarily a ceremonial task. A joint session of the Congress, presided over by the vice president, meets to count the electoral vote as certified by the fifty states. The president told Vice President Mike Pence that, as he presided over the proceeding, he should send the electoral votes back to the contested states so they could recount them in his favor. He insisted that the states wanted to do this (they did not). This was pure nonsense, of course, but there was another long shot option that might come into play if the president's most ardent supporters in the U.S. Congress had their way.

There was a procedure through which the electors of a specific state could be challenged. This required a member of the House and a member of the Senate to object to including that state's vote in the count. Where this might occur, the House and Senate must meet in their separate chambers to debate the challenge for two hours. Then each house must vote to support or reject the challenge. For a state's vote to be rejected, majorities in both the House and Senate must support the challenge. President Trump's strongest Republican supporters in the House and Senate planned to challenge the electoral vote in each of the most closely contested states won by Biden. If successful, these challenges could hold Biden's electoral vote below the 270-vote majority required to be declared the winner. If that were to happen, the presidential election would be decided by the U.S. House of Representatives. Each state delegation would have one vote. While the Democrats did hold a majority of seats in the House, the majority of state delegations were controlled by Republicans. This meant that, were the election to go to the House, Donald Trump would likely win a majority of the state delegations and be declared president for another four years.

In anticipation of January 6 and the counting of the electoral vote by the Congress, President Trump pulled out all the stops. Claiming that it was "statistically impossible" that he had lost the presidential election, Trump urged his supporters to come to the U.S. Capitol and interrupt what is typically a ceremonial joint session. "Peter Navarro releases 36-page report alleging election fraud 'more than sufficient' to swing victory to Trump," the president tweeted. "A great report by Peter. Statistically impossible to have lost the 2020 Election. Big protest in D.C. on January 6th. Be there, will be wild!" The most vehement pro-Trump Republicans in the House and several in the Senate made it clear that they could be counted on to challenge and disrupt the counting of the electoral vote.[32]

The president had to be very pleased to see the crowd gathered for his "Save America" rally in front of the White House at 11:00 a.m. on January 6. Thousands of Trump loyalists and various white supremacy and anti-government extremists had eagerly gathered in answer to President Trump's invitation to come to Washington, DC, to "save America." The rally began with speeches from the president's sons Eric and Donald Trump Jr. and then his lawyer, Rudy Giuliani. The president himself spoke at about 11:50 a.m. Giuliani called for "trial by combat." Donald Trump Jr. warned the Congress that "we are coming for you." President Trump was at his bombastic best with an inflammatory speech that fired up the crowd. He raged against the "radical Democrats" and the "fake news media," who had conspired to steal the election from him and his patriotic supporters. He urged the crowd to "stop the steal." A passage of his speech clearly directed his followers to go to Capitol Hill. "And after this, we're going to walk down there, and I'll be there with you, we're going to walk down . . . to the Capitol and we are going to cheer on our brave senators and congressmen and women," Trump told the crowd. "And we're probably not going to be cheering so much for some of them. Because you'll never take back our country with weakness. You have to show strength and you have to be strong."

The president had tried to persuade Vice President Pence that he had the authority to simply refuse to accept the electoral votes from the contested states. At the rally on January 6, he told his listeners, "I hope Mike is going to do the right thing. . . . Because if Mike Pence does the right thing, we win the election." He insisted to his supporters that Vice President Pence had the authority to send it back to the states for a revote. "States want to revote. The States got defrauded. They were given false information. They voted on it. Now they want to recertify. They want it back. All Vice-President Pence has to do is send it back to the States to recertify, and we become president, and you are the happiest people."[33] All of this was pure nonsense. The last prayer of a desperate mind that had long ago lost any contact with the truth. But it worked on his audience and made them all the more determined to "save America." Trump concluded, "Our country has had enough. We will not take it anymore, and that's what this is all about. To use a favorite term that all of you people really came up with, we will stop the steal." When he was finished with his hour-long incitement, his supporters headed for the U.S. Capitol Building as instructed.

At 1:00 p.m., lawmakers had gathered for a joint session in the House of Representatives chamber to count Electoral College votes. At 1:10 p.m., rioters begin grappling with police on the Capitol's steps. It had come to this. Amid American flags and Trump 2020 posters, the U.S. Capitol was under siege. Soon members of the House and Senate were evacuated from the House chamber. At 2:24 p.m., Trump tweeted, "Mike Pence didn't have the courage to do what should have been done to protect our Country and our Constitution, giving States a chance to certify a corrected set of facts, not the fraudulent or inaccurate ones which they were asked to previously certify. USA demands the truth!" By 2:33 p.m., rioters had crossed the National Statuary Hall, which separates the chambers, heading for the House and Senate. The Capitol Building had been overtaken by rioters.[34] Among the sights seen by Americans on their television screens were a man walking the halls of Congress carrying a Confederate flag, banners proclaiming white supremacy and anti-government extremism, and the hateful imagery of a man wearing an anti-Semitic "Camp Auschwitz" sweatshirt. A makeshift noose had been erected outside. Presumably this was a symbol, but who knows? Some of the rioters were shouting, "Hang Mike Pence!" This is what "Saving America" looked like. It was not a sight welcomed by any patriotic American, or so one would like to think.

One must note that not all who invaded the Capitol on January 6 were merely Trump supporters. Extremist groups, including the pro-Trump anti-government Oath Keepers (many of whom are retired police or military), the Three Percenters (a loose anti-government network and part of the militia movement), Q-Anon (believers in a conspiracy theory that all Democrats in the government are child abusers and are about to be arrested, as President Trump and federal law enforcement would shut down the transition and lock them all up, etc.), and other white nationalist and white supremacist groups, were prominent among those attacking the Article I branch of the federal government on this fateful day.

As the assault on the Capitol proceeded and members of the House and Senate were rushed to safety or hiding under desks and the vice president was escorted to safety, what was the president of the United States doing? As we have seen, President Trump was tweeting his displeasure with Vice President Pence's refusal to do as he had instructed him: "Mike Pence didn't have the courage to do what should have been done to protect our Country and our Constitution, giving States a chance to certify a corrected set of facts, not the fraudulent or inaccurate ones which they were asked to previously certify. USA demands the truth!"[35] Capitol Police, assisted by DC Police and eventually eleven hundred National Guard troops, were ultimately able to restore order.

In all, five deaths occurred during the violent assault on the Capitol. As rioters were forcing their way toward the House chamber where members of Congress were sheltering in place, a sworn U.S. Capitol Police employee discharged his service weapon, striking and killing an adult female. In addition to the woman shot by Capitol Police, two men and one woman died in separate medical emergencies. A U.S. Capitol Police officer also died due to injuries sustained in the attack, thus bringing the total number of fatalities to five.[36] It could have been much worse, as some rioters were shouting that Mike Pence should be hung and others sought out various congressional leaders for capture or worse. Order would finally be returned, and as a stunned nation tried to comprehend what it had just observed, the joint session of Congress reconvened to certify the electoral vote at 8:00 p.m. that evening.

In the vote Wednesday evening, January 6, following what had amounted to a violent insurrection that afternoon by President Trump and his various supporters, 6 Republicans in the Senate and 121 in the House backed objections to certifying Arizona's electoral outcome, and 7 Senate Republicans and 138 House Republicans supported an objection to certifying Pennsylvania's electoral outcome. The lawmakers who made these objections, even though they were completely unfounded, served only to further amplify lies about a rigged election. These lawmakers in essence co-conspired with the president to overturn a free and fair election. Neither the Arizona nor the Pennsylvania objections obtained a majority of votes in either chamber, so both failed. Other challenges had been promised by the president's "co-conspirators" in the "big lie," but the events of the day thankfully prompted a number of Republicans to drop their previous challenges. Still, the decision by so many Republicans (145 of them) to persist in making any bogus challenges after the attack on the Capitol suggested that they were shockingly comfortable undermining the democratic process. Congress had, as was inevitable from the beginning, certified President-elect Joe Biden as the winner of the election. The electoral vote (306 for Biden and 232 for Trump) was finally made official.

Donald Trump did not succeed in overturning the election results, but he did succeed in making history of a very different sort. Donald Trump's role in inciting the January 6 Capitol riot led to his being impeached for a second time and to the first impeachment trial of a president after leaving office. Why hold an impeachment trial after the president had left office? Many said he needed to be held accountable for what he had done. More important to others, if the Senate voted to convict Trump, it could then invoke the constitutionally created sanction of "disqualification to hold and enjoy any Office of honor, Trust or Profit under the United States." This would mean no 2024 presidential campaign or comeback attempt for Donald Trump.

On Wednesday, January 13, one week after the assault on the Capitol, the House began debating impeachment. After a brisk two-hour debate, the House voted to impeach Trump on a single article of "incitement to insurrection." The vote, 232–197, included ten Republicans crossing party lines to support the article of impeachment. This drama would play itself out in the early days of the next administration. From the get-go, no one could reasonably expect a conviction in the Senate. There was absolutely no chance of that happening. And for his part, President-elect Joe Biden would have other pressing matters occupying his time and constant attention after January 20, 2021.

Donald Trump entered January 2020, the beginning of his last year as president, just as the United States recorded its first confirmed case of COVID-19. Not to worry, he insisted, his administration had the virus "totally under control." On his final full day in office, January 19, 2021, the pandemic's U.S. death toll had eclipsed four hundred thousand, and the loss of lives was accelerating. President-elect Joe Biden, who would be sworn in the next day, did something that President Trump would never think of doing. He took part in an evening ceremony near the Lincoln Memorial in Washington to honor the four hundred thousand dead. The bell at the Washington National Cathedral tolled four hundred times to remember the dead. Other cities around the United States observed tributes as well.

As president, Donald Trump had never seemed to realize that he was uniquely positioned and expected to comfort Americans in a time of difficulty. Not that this was his nature. He used his pulpit for other purposes. He used it to promote and comfort himself, not to comfort others He invested more time trying to manipulate public perceptions about the pandemic for his political benefit than he did fighting the virus itself. He downplayed the threat, rejected scientific expertise, and fanned the conflicts ignited by the pandemic. To be sure, the COVID-19 pandemic would have brought tragedy and suffering to Americans under the best of circumstances. From January 2020 to January 2021, it had infected over twenty-four million Americans, including President Trump and members of his family, and it had killed more than four hundred thousand Americans. Under the best of circumstances, with a more coherent and science-driven national response, fewer would have been infected, and fewer would have died. But the United States did not enjoy the best of circumstances. By any measure, 2020 was a year of monumental failure for the United States. To put it bluntly, too much of the pandemic damage had been self-inflicted.

Conclusion: It Didn't Have to Be This Bad

The worst part of the coronavirus pandemic was not how much of a surprise it was to most Americans but how utterly predictable it was and how unprepared the U.S. government had been to handle the crisis. This lack of preparation was, as we have seen in our summary of pandemic-related events throughout 2020, somewhat of a surprise to many. Hadn't the Global Health Security (GHS) Index rated the United States as the best prepared nation to deal with a public health emergency? Hadn't both the Bush and Obama administrations made significant progress in upgrading American planning and preparedness for a pandemic? This progress combined with the things we had been able to learn from a rapid succession of global health episodes (i.e., H1N1, Ebola, and Zika) would, as previously noted, show us where our pandemic planning was incomplete and give us opportunities to keep improving it. We knew what needed to be done. The sad truth of the matter is that we just did not do it.

What needed to be done was well known when Donald Trump entered office in January 2017. This knowledge was based on the experiences and scientific insights that had been gained by the previous two administrations. There were, as we have seen, obvious and straightforward items to be pursued as the planning process continued. Among the most basic of things that a national response to a pandemic required, we emphasized the following: First, it was essential to ensure that national leadership during any pandemic scenario be upgraded and prioritized. The federal government, we noted, needed to present a unified message to guide state and local officials and to responsibly manage the American public's questions and concerns during the crisis. Second, the coordination of all federal agencies needed to interact smoothly and efficiently during an unfolding pandemic crisis. This meant making sure that all public health agencies, especially the CDC, provided scientifically sound directives to guide the actions of state and local governments and responders. We noted that all these things needed to be done in a timely and coordinated fashion and with detail, clarity, and a unified message. Third, it meant informing the public with a consistent and science-based strategy. Improving public awareness with accurate and timely information was said to be a priority of the utmost importance. This federal "leadership" need was based on the understanding that while a multistate effort would be needed in response to a pandemic, this effort needed to have direction and be consistent from state to state. States and citizens alike would be best served by a well-organized federal effort to inform and guide all actors, public and private.

The other needs to be met were also very obvious. These included more consistent support for the research and development of vaccines, therapeutics, and diagnostics. It was of critical importance to invest the resources and the effort required to replenish the stockpiles of countermeasure and response supplies that first responders would need during a public health emergency. It was important that the federal government be prepared to be aggressively active in assisting the states and localities as their systems became overwhelmed and their supplies came up short. On the international level, it was regarded as essential for the United States to continue and to enhance its coordination with other nations in ongoing research and to improve the coordination of global response activities. Each of these needs would require sustained and persistent work to ensure that the United States could respond effectively to a pandemic.

There was, it will be recalled, a pandemic playbook that outlined these needs and the recommended steps to be taken to meet them. This pandemic playbook, passed down from President Barack Obama to President Donald Trump, was an important planning document. It laid out the decisions to be made and the agencies to be mobilized in a public health disaster. Its stated goal was to prepare the nation for the worst global pandemic in one hundred years. Most importantly, the document stressed the need for a national public health response coordinated by the federal government. As our narrative has shown, that never happened in 2020.

None of the needs emphasized in over a decade of pandemic planning would be met.

The United States was well prepared, but it had one of the worst outcomes because its strong capabilities were squandered when they were most needed. The nation's leaders, beginning with President Trump, ignored warnings about the dire consequences of leaving the states to fend for themselves. President Trump certainly never understood the central role of the federal government. Fifty states running in fifty different directions was, to put it succinctly, a recipe for failure. Absent a national effort and a coherent national strategy, states were forced to compete with one another to purchase scarce medical supplies. In the absence of detailed federal guidelines, states imposed a hodgepodge of lockdown policies, only to have some of these plans undermined by politicians, including and especially the president.

There were other longer-term failures that also combined to make the situation worse than it needed to be. Despite more than a decade of scientific warnings about the specific threat posed by coronaviruses, the government and drug companies allowed research on a potential coronavirus vaccine to be shelved for three years instead of testing it in human trials. Despite more than a decade of warnings about a serious global pandemic, funding for public health had been steadily cut for more than a decade. Indeed, with respect to public health concerns generally, the nation had for some time not prioritized being prepared for a crisis. But, above all else, our summary of the 2020 response to COVID-19 suggests that the greatest failure was one of leadership. It was, we might say, the leadership dimension that was the most lethal of the fuels that allowed the pandemic fires to burn out of control.

President Trump, as we have seen, dismissed the advice of public health experts, downplayed the seriousness of the pandemic, and deliberately undermined confidence in our public health agencies. It will be remembered that the president told journalist Bob Woodward, as recounted in the book *Rage*, that he played down the pandemic because he did not want to panic the American public. Leaders of other countries worked to inform and unite their citizens behind the idea of collective sacrifice. They were better prepared than Americans, one might suggest, to cooperate on the various measures necessary to contain the spread of the virus.

The president, and many Republican governors and supporters, politicized the pandemic and divided the public. Debates over masking, social distancing, stay-at-home orders, and every other effort to contain the spread of the virus led to poor decisions by government and the American people. These poor decisions fed the beast and primed the nation for a pandemic disaster that would indeed become much worse than it needed to be. Various experts have opined that many American deaths (perhaps as many as two hundred thousand) could have been avoided with earlier policy interventions and more robust federal coordination and leadership. We have seen in our 2020 narrative that U.S. fatalities remained disproportionately high throughout the pandemic when compared to even other high-mortality countries. We have seen that when measured by deaths per one hundred thousand population, the US mortality rate is fifty times higher than Japan's and more than twice as high as Canada's. We saw insufficient testing, a lack of national mask mandates, political interference with public health guidelines, miscommunication, public confusion, partisan division, and the lack of a coordinated national response put the United States at the top of the global coronavirus death toll.

As has been noted several times throughout the course of this narrative, there would have been tragic outcomes even under the best of circumstances. No pandemic plan or national strategy, however perfectly implemented, would have prevented all the ravages that a pandemic brings with it. But the failures of our national leadership during the first year of the COVID-19 pandemic did make things much worse. Three general failures characterized the Trump-imposed confusion and ineptitude that destroyed the nation's capacity to act effectively to control the virus. These were three big failures that gave birth to all the assorted little failures to come as the year 2020 wore the nation down.

President Trump failed to recognize and communicate the early signs of danger, he refused to lead a fast ramp-up and national response when he did recognize the danger, and he persisted throughout the crisis to spread the misinformation and confusion that inhibited our ability to implement public health measures that have been proven lifesavers. When he left office on January 20, 2021, the nation had not so much as begun to truly address the pandemic with a national strategy.

The day President Joe Biden assumed office, he walked into a pandemic still raging out of control, killing thousands more people in the United States each day. The United States, with just a little more than 4 percent of the world's population, had accounted for 20 percent of the worldwide COVID-19 fatalities from January 21, 2020, to January 20, 2021. The U.S. death toll had reached 400,000. During the first ten days of the new administration, over 38,000 more Americans died. Projections were that the death toll would reach over 500,000 by the end of February and more than 600,000 by the end of March. On the very day of the Biden inauguration, 4,133 more American COVID-19 deaths were recorded.

Two very effective vaccines against the virus that causes COVID-19 were approved for emergency use in the United States about a month before President Biden took office, but by most indicators, the distribution of these vaccines was not very well organized. According to various media reports, one of the biggest shocks that the Biden team had to deal with during the transition period was what they saw as the complete lack of a vaccine distribution strategy under the Trump administration. This caused them great concern about the vaccine rollout. On almost every front of the pandemic response, the Biden administration would have to essentially start from square one because there simply was no plan in place.

President Biden began his administration with rolling out his national strategy for addressing the pandemic crisis. A full year after the first case of the virus had been confirmed, the United States finally had what it had needed on day one, a national strategy. As a candidate during the election campaign, Biden promised that he would implement a massive federal response to address the coronavirus pandemic. This would include free testing and an aggressive vaccine rollout. He promised that his administration would ensure that one hundred million Americans would be vaccinated in the first one hundred days. He was also determined to address the resources needed to help schools reopen. He promised to see that small businesses, families, and marginalized populations received the assistance they needed. He would seek to implement mask mandates nationwide by working with mayors and governors to set up local orders and asking individual Americans to wear masks when they were around people outside their household. He would seek to provide clear, evidence-based public health guidance about social distancing and make sure the CDC gave communities clear guidance on when measures such as school closures, stay-at-home orders, or restaurant restrictions needed to be implemented or could be ended. He also felt it essential to provide emergency funding for state and local governments, schools, and small businesses so they could get back on their feet.

In his first days in office, President Biden quickly expanded U.S. defenses to prevent and respond to future pandemics. He restored the White House National Security Council Directorate for Global Health Security and Biodefense and rejoined the World Health Organization. He also relaunched the pathogen-tracking program called PREDICT. It was a heavy lift, and the details of meeting each of these objectives were complex, perhaps even mind-numbing. But this is the work of government, when all is said and done. Joe Biden entered the presidency determined to see that the work of government would be done expertly and efficiently.

The year 2021 would be another COVID-19 year. The nation would have a long way to go before the coronavirus might be contained and the crisis under control. The failures of 2020 meant that 2021 would be filled with challenges that were still expanding because of opportunities missed. The path to normal, or a new normal, was still a good way off. The task of vaccinating the population would take months to reach the point where herd immunity might be achieved. New strains of the virus were circulating, and some of these were thought to be more contagious. One or more of these new stains might soon become the dominant strain in the United States. It was thought that the vaccines being administered would provide protection against them, but there were enough unknowns about that to be a bit wary. By the end of the summer 2021, the U.S. death toll would top 650,000, and some were predicting it would reach 800,000 by the end of the year.

Still, though there were difficult days ahead, there was reason for hope. The United States seemed to have leadership that was finally moving forward with a national strategy. As one reflects on the year 2020, on the first cases of a new coronavirus infection in the Hubei Province of China, the spread of that virus across the globe, the American experience of that virus, and ultimately on the incredible failure of the United States to respond effectively to a global pandemic, one thing above all stands out. As horrific and deadly as a pandemic can be, it is even more horrific to see public officials amplify that horror and death through their ineptitude or corruption.

Why did Donald Trump refuse to mobilize the resources of this nation to implement a plan or national strategy for addressing the pandemic? Why did he play it down? Why did he call it a "hoax" designed by his political enemies and the media? Why did he ignore his public health experts, contradict them, and ultimately discredit them in the eyes of his many supporters? Why did he incite protests against state stay-at-home orders? Why did he criticize governors who acted prudently to implement them? Why did he politicize a public health crisis? Why did he stop even talking about the pandemic after the November 3 election? Why did he seek to make the overturning of a free and fair election his only priority in the last two months he was in office? Most importantly, why did so many Republican governors and other officeholders and his supporters in the media and among the public support him without question in all of these things?

The answers to each of these questions will undoubtedly be the topics of many books to come. The one thing that is clear, whether Donald Trump or any other elected leader did what they did because they were acting out of political expediency, corruption, incompetence, or fear, the 2020 "great American fail" was first and foremost a failure of leadership.

The leadership factor is often why even the best of plans fail. Absent any planning or preparedness for a crisis, even great leaders will fail. The combination of no national strategy, no commitment to preparedness, and a historic leadership failure was the perfect storm that destroyed everything in its path. That was 2020 in the United States. It was a perfect storm that gave birth to the greatest failure in American history. That must be understood, and it must never be forgotten or excused.

In the years to come, and as more details of the events of 2020 in the United States become known, there will be more detailed analysis of both the COVID-19 pandemic and the U.S. response to it. But the experience of the year 2020 in the United States needs to be understood by those who lived through it and by the generations who will only read or hear about it in the years to come. There will be future pandemics. There will be future global crises that will equal and, in all likelihood, surpass the horror of the COVID-19 pandemic. When these future events occur, our preparations for them will in all probability be inadequate. Even if they are not, it must always be remembered that even the very best of plans are not perfect.

But let it be hoped that no future generation will suffer through a leadership failure anywhere near as devastating as the United States did in 2020. As we observed early on in this narrative, even with the proper reliance on science and the availability of expertise to guide them, political leaders will find themselves tested to the limit of their abilities in a public health crisis. Let us hope that the United States will never again find its leaders during such a crisis to be of such limited ability as was the case in the year 2020.

Notes

Prologue

1. Pilkington, E. (2021). "'An Unmitigated Disaster': America's Year of COVID." *The Guardian*, January 18, 2021. https://www.theguardian.com/world/2021/jan/18/america-year-of-covid-coronavirus-deaths-cases (accessed February 1, 2021).

2. Ibid.

3. Schneider, R. (2009). "H5N1 Planning Concerns for Local Governments." *Journal of Emergency Management* 7, no. 1 (January–February): 65–70.

4. Schneider, R. (2018). *When Science and Politics Collide: The Public Interest at Risk*. Santa Barbara, CA: Praeger.

Chapter One

1. Johns Hopkins.org. (2020). "What Is Coronavirus?" https://www.hopkinsmedicine.org/health/conditions-and-diseases/coronavirus (accessed May 11, 2020).

2. Ibid.

3. Readfearn, G. (2020). "How Did Coronavirus Start and Where Did It Come From?" *The Guardian*, April 28, 2020. https://www.theguardian.com/world/2020/apr/28/how-did-the-coronavirus-start-where-did-it-come-from-how-did-it-spread-humans-was-it-really-bats-pangolins-wuhan-animal-market (accessed May 11, 2020).

4. Zelicoff, A.P., and Bellomo, M. (2005). *Are We Ready for the Next Plague?* New York: American Management Association.

5. Schneider, R.O. (2018). *When Science and Politics Collide: The Public Interest at Risk*. Santa Barbara, CA: Praeger.

6. Lanese, N. (2020). "What Is a Coronavirus?" *Live Science*, February 7, 2020. https://www.livescience.com/what-are-coronaviruses.html (accessed May 11, 2020).

7. Ledford, H. (2020). "How Does COVID-19 Kill? Uncertainty Is Hampering Doctors' Ability to Choose Treatments." *Nature*, April 9, 2020. https://www.nature.com/articles/d41586-020-01056-7 (accessed May 12, 2020).

8. Mundell, E.J. (2020). "Odds of Hospitalization, Death with COVID-19 Rise Steadily with Age: Study." *U.S. News and World Report*, March 31, 2020. https://www.usnews.com/news/health-news/articles/2020-03-30/odds-of-hospitalization-death-with-covid-19-rise-steadily-with-age-study (accessed May 17, 2020).

9. Centers for Disease Control and Prevention. (2020). "CDC Updates, Expands List of People at Risk of Severe COVID-19 Illness." June 25, 2020. https://www.cdc.gov/media/releases/2020/p0625-update-expands-covid-19.html (accessed July 19, 2020).

10. World Health Organization. (2020). "WHO Director-General's Remarks at the Media Briefing on 2019-nCoV on 11 February 2020." https://www.who.int/dg/speeches/detail/who-director-general-s-remarks-at-the-media-briefing-on-2019-ncov-on-11-february-2020 (accessed May 17, 2020).

11. Kickok, K. (2020). "What Is a Pandemic?" Live Science, March 3, 2020. https://www.livescience.com/pandemic.html (accessed May 18, 2020).

12. Ibid.

13. Bristow, Nancy K. (2012). *American Pandemic.* Oxford, UK: Oxford University Press.

14. Quammen, David. (2012). *Spillover: Animal Infections and the Next Human Pandemic.* New York: W. W. Norton & Company.

15. Taylor, Steven. (2019). *The Psychology of Pandemics: Preparing for the Next Outbreak of Infectious Disease.* New Castle, UK: Cambridge Scholars Publishing.

16. Johns Hopkins Coronavirus Research Center. (2020). "Mortality Analysis." https://coronavirus.jhu.edu/data/mortality (accessed May 20, 2020).

Chapter Two

1. ABC News. (2020). "George W. Bush in 2005: 'If We Wait for a Pandemic to Appear, It Will Be Too Late to Prepare.'" April 5, 2020. https://abcnews.go.com/Politics/george-bush-2005-wait-pandemic-late-prepare/story?id=69979013 (accessed May 25, 2020).

2. Ibid.

3. White House Archives. (2005). "National Strategy for Pandemic Influenza." November 1, 2005. https://georgewbush-whitehouse.archives.gov/homeland/pandemic-influenza.html (accessed May 25, 2020).

4. Walsh, B. (2017). "The World Is Not Ready for the Next Pandemic." *Time*, May 15, 2017.

5. Gillian, K.S., Blendon, R.J., Bekheit, J.D., and Lubell, K. (2010). "The Public's Response to the 2009 H1N1 Virus." *New England Journal of Medicine.* http://www.nejm.org/doi/full/10.1056/NEJMp1005102 (accessed May 26, 2020).

6. Newsstand. (2020). "Six Years Ago, President Obama Predicted the Need for Quick Pandemic Response." May 25, 2020. http://newsstand7.com/2020/04

/12/six-years-ago-president-obama-predicted-the-need-for-quick-pandemic -response/ (accessed May 25, 2020).

7. Schneider, R.O. (2009). "H5N1 Planning Concerns for Local Governments." *Journal of Emergency Management* 7, no 1: 65–70.

8. Mossad, S.B. (2007). "Influenza Update 2007–2008: Vaccine Advances, Pandemic Preparation." *Cleveland Clinic Journal of Medicine* 74, no. 12: 884–894.

9. World Health Organization. (n.d.). "Influenza." http://www.who.int/csr /disease/avian_influenza/en/ (accessed May 28, 2020).

10. Schneider, R.O. (2018). *When Science and Politics Collide: The Public Interest at Risk.* Santa Barbara, CA: Praeger.

11. Gregor, M. (2006). *Bird Flu: A Virus of Our Own Hatching.* New York: Lancaster Books.

12. Barry, J.M. (2005). *The Great Influenza.* New York: Penguin Books.

13. Ibid.

14. Gregor, *Bird Flu.*

15. Rivera, R. (2006). "Prepare for Pandemic, Localities Are Warned." *Washington Post*, February 25, 2006.

16. Schneider, "H5N1 Planning Concerns for Local Governments."

17. Cooper, K.E. (2007). "The Shadows of Pandemic." In *Global Pandemics*, edited by C. Mari. New York: H. W. Wilson.

18. Disease Control Priorities Project. (2008). "Public Health Surveillance: The Best Weapon to Avert Epidemics." https://www.scribd.com/document /55423821/Dcpp-Surveillance (accessed September 11, 2008).

19. Greenwood, J. (2015). "How Prepared Are We for Avian Flu?" The Hill, July 29, 2015. http://thehill.com/blogs/congress-blog/healthcare/249506-how -prepared-are-we-for-avian-flu (accessed May 10, 2020).

20. Ibid.

21. Gregor, *Bird Flu.*

22. Ibid.

23. Ibid.

24. Boin, A., Hart, P., Stern, E., and Sundelius, B. (2005). *The Politics of Crisis Management: Public Leadership under Pressure.* Cambridge, UK: Cambridge University Press.

25. American Public Health Association. (2007). "APHA Opinion Survey on Public Health Preparedness." www.nphw.org/2007/pg_toos_poll.htm (accessed September 23, 2007).

26. Fischhoff, B. (1995). "Risk Perception and Communication Unplugged: Twenty Years of Process." *Risk Analysis* 15, no. 2: 137–145.

27. Ibid.

28. Thomas, J., Dasgupta, N., and Martinot, A. (2007). "Ethics in a Pandemic: A Survey of the State Pandemic Influenza Plans." *American Journal of Public Health* 97: 526–531.

29. Steenhuysen, J. (2009). "U.S. Health Department Response to H1N1 Mixed: Study." Reuters, July 7, 2009. http://www.reuters.com/article/us-flu-usa -idUSTRE56669020090707 (accessed June 3, 2020).

30. Ibid.

31. Gillian et al., "The Public's Response."

32. Association of State and Territorial Health Officials. (2010). "Addressing Policy Barriers to Effective Public Health Response in the H5N1 Influenza Pandemic: Project Report to the Centers for Disease Control and Prevention." https://astho.org/Programs/Infectious-Disease/H1N1/H1N1-Barriers-Project-Report-Final-hi-res/ (accessed June 3, 2020).

33. Ibid.

34. Walsh, "The World Is Not Ready for the Next Pandemic."

35. Ikejezie, J., Shapiro, C.N., Kim, J., Chiu, M., Almiron, M., Ugarte, C., Espinal, M.A., and Aldighieri, S. (2016). "Zika Virus Transmission—Region of the Americas, May 15, 2015–December 15, 2016." *Morbidity and Mortality Weekly Report* 66, no 12: 329–334. https://doi.org/10.15585/mmwr.mm6612a4 (accessed June 4, 2020).

36. Greer, S.L. (2016). "Political Fights behind Uneven U.S. Zika Response." *Scientific American*, September 6, 2016. https://www.scientificamerican.com/article/political-fights-behind-uneven-u-s-zika-response/ (accessed June 4, 2020).

37. Ibid.

38. Ibid.

39. Department of Homeland Security. (2014). "DHS Has Not Effectively Managed Pandemic Personal Protective Equipment and Medical Countermeasures." https://www.oig.dhs.gov/assets/Mgmt/2014/OIG_14-129_Aug14.pdf (accessed April 29, 2017).

40. Shinkman, P.D. (2017). "If a Pandemic Hits, the U.S. Isn't Ready." *U.S. News and World Report*, May 4, 2017. https://www.usnews.com/news/health-care-news/articles/2017-05-04/us-falling-short-on-pandemic-prevention-study-says (accessed June4, 2020).

41. Medscape. (2016). "The World Is Not Prepared for Pandemics." November 15, 2016. http://www.medscape.com/viewarticle/871802 (accessed June 4, 2020).

42. Karlawish, J. (2020). "A Pandemic Plan Was in Place. Trump Abandoned It—and Science—in the Face of COVID-19." First Opinion, STAT, May 17, 2020. www.statnews.com/2020/05.17/the=art-of-the-pandemic-how-donald-trump=walked-the-u=s-into-the-covid-19-era/ (accessed June 5, 2020).

43. Ibid.

44. *Playbook for Early Response to High-Consequence Emerging Infectious Disease Threats and Biological Incidents*. Washington, DC: Executive Office of the President of the United States. https://brian.carnell.com/wp-content/uploads/2020/03/WH-Pandemic-Playbook.pdf.

45. Ibid.

46. Ibid

47. Lewis, M. (2018). *The Fifth Risk: Undoing Democracy*. New York: W. W. Norton & Company.

48. Koblentz. G.D., and Morra, N.M. (2017). "Pandemics, Personnel, and Politics: How the Trump Administration Is Leaving Us Vulnerable to the Next Outbreak." *Global Biodefense*, April 6, 2017.

49. Ibid.

50. Ibid.

Chapter Three

1. History.com Editors. (2009). "Galileo Is Accused of Heresy." November 13, 2009. https://www.history.com/this-day-in-history/galileo-is-accused-of-heresy (accessed June 10, 2020).

2. de Tocqueville, Alexis. (1966). *Democracy in America*. Translated by George Lawrence. New York: Harper and Row.

3. Ibid.

4. Bella, R.N., Madsen, R., Sullivan, W.M., Swidler, A., and Tipton, S.M. (2007). *Habits of Heart: Individualism and Commitment in American Life*. Berkeley, CA: University of California Press.

5. Gans, H.J. (1988). *Middle American Individualism: Popular Participation and Liberal Democracy*. New York: Oxford University Press.

6. Hofstadter, R. (1963). *Anti-Intellectualism in American Life*. New York: Vintage Books.

7. Ibid.

8. Bauerlein, M. (2008). *The Dumbest Generation: How the Digital Age Stupefies Young Americans and Jeopardizes Our Future*. New York: Jeremy P. Tarcher/Penguin.

9. Pew Research Center. (2019). "Democrats More Supportive Than Republicans of Federal Spending for Scientific Research." September 4, 2019. https://www.pewresearch.org/fact-tank/2019/09/04/democrats-more-supportive-than-republicans-of-federal-spending-for-scientific-research/ (accessed June 16, 2020).

10. Ibid.

11. Doherty, C. (2014). "7 Things to Know about Polarization in America." Pew Research Center. http://www.pewresearch.org/fact-tank/2014/06/12/7-things-to-know-about-polarizatioin-in-america/ (accessed June 16, 2020).

12. Ibid.

13. Hetherington, M.J., and Weller, J.D. (2009). *Authoritarianism and Polarization in American Politics*. New York: Cambridge University Press.

14. Otto, S. (2016). *The War on Science*. Minneapolis, MN: Milkweed Editions.

15. Ibid.

16. Ibid.

17. Schneider, R.O. (2018). *When Science and Politics Collide: The Public Interest at Risk*. Santa Barbara, CA: Praeger.

18. Silver, H. J. (2006). "Science and Politics: The Uneasy Relationship." *Footnotes* 34, no. 2. https://www.asanet.org/sites/default/files/fn_2006_02.pdf (accessed June 17, 2020).

19. B. D. (2013). "A Failed Experiment." *The Economist*, September 19, 2013. https://www.economist.com/democracy-in-america/2013/09/19/a-failed-experiment (accessed June 17, 2020).

20. Oreskes, N., and Conway, E. (2010). *Merchants of Doubt*. New York: Bloomsbury Press.

21. Ibid.

22. Mann, M.E. (2016). "I'm a Scientist Who Has Gotten Death Threats. I Fear What May Happen under Trump." *Washington Post*, December 16, 2016.

23. Maasen, S., and Weingart, P. (2005). "What's New in Scientific Advice to Politics?" In *Democratization of Expertise: Exploring Novel Forms of Scientific Advice in Political Decision-Making*, edited by S. Maasen and P. Weingart, 1–19. New York: Springer Business and Media.

24. Ibid.

25. Silver, "Science and Politics."

26. Cook, J., and Lewandowsky, S. (2016). "Rational Irrationality: Modeling Climate Change Belief Polarization Using Bayesian Networks." *Topics in Cognitive Science* 8, no. 1: 160–179.

27. Ibid.

28. Otto, *The War on Science*.

29. Ibid.

30. Hale, T. (2018). "Here Are Just A Few Of the Ridiculous Anti-Science Things That President Donald Trump Actually Believes." *IFL Science*, November 23, 2018. https://www.iflscience.com/policy/here-are-just-a-few-of-the-ridiculous-antiscience-things-that-president-donald-trump-actually-believes (accessed June 19, 2020).

31. Slisco, A. (2020). "Fauci Blames Anti-Science Bias for People Not Following COVID-19 Rules." *Newsweek*, June 18, 2020. https://www.newsweek.com/fauci-blames-anti-science-bias-people-not-following-covid-19-rules-1512019 (accessed June 22, 2020).

32. Funk, C., Hefferon, M., Kennedy, B., and Johnson, C. (2019). "Trust and Mistrust in Americans' Views of Scientific Experts." Pew Research Center, August 2, 2019. https://www.pewresearch.org/science/2019/08/02/partisanship-influences-views-on-the-role-and-value-of-scientific-experts-in-policy-debates/(accessed June 22, 2020).

33. Kuntzman, G. (2017). "Trump's War on Science Continues with EPA Firings." *New York Daily News*, May 8, 2017. https://www.nydailynews.com/news/national/trump-war-science-continues-epa-firings-article-1.3147062 (accessed June 26, 2020).

34. Ibid.

35. Parker, L., and Welch, C. (2017). "3 Things You Need to Know about the Science Rebellion against Trump." *National Geographic*, January 27, 2017. https://www.nationalgeographic.com/news/2017/01/scientists-march-on-washington-national-parks-twitter-war-climate-science-donald-trump/ (accessed June 26, 2020).

36. Ibid.

37. Walsh, B. (2017). "The World Is Not Ready for the Next Pandemic." *Time*, May 15, 2017.

38. Koblentz, G.D., and Morra, N.M. (2017). "Pandemics. Personnel, and Politics: How the Trump Administration Is Leaving Us Vulnerable to the Next Outbreak." *Global Biodefense*, April 6, 2017.

39. Ibid.

40. Budryk, Z. (2020). "WHO Chief Warns Leaders against 'Politicizing' Pandemic." The Hill, June 22, 2020. https://thehill.com/policy/healthcare/503863 -who-chief-warns-leaders-against-politicizing-pandemic (accessed June 26, 2020).

Chapter Four

1. Wolfe, M. (2018). *Fire and Fury: Inside the Trump White House.* New York: McMillan Publishing Group.

2. Ibid.

3. Anonymous. (2019). *A Warning.* New York: Hachette Book Group, Inc.

4. Ibid.

5. Markowitz, D. (2020). "Trump Is Lying More Than Ever: Just Look at the Data." *Forbes*, May 5, 2020. https://www.forbes.com/sites/davidmarkowitz /2020/05/05/trump-is-lying-more-than-ever-just-look-at-the-data/# 69a12ab31e17 (accessed July 1, 2020).

6. *Washington Post.* (2019). *The Mueller Report.* New York: Scribner.

7. Baumgaertner, E., and Rainey, J. (2020). "Trump Administration Ended Pandemic Early-Warning Program to Detect Coronaviruses." *Los Angeles Times*, April 2, 2020. https://www.latimes.com/science/story/2020-04-02/coronavirus -trump-pandemic-program-viruses-detection (accessed July 3, 2020).

8. Ibid.

9. Bolton, J. (2020). *The Room Where It Happened.* New York: Simon and Schuster.

10. Ibid.

11. Bergengruen, V., and Hennigan, W.J. (2020). "Doomed from the Start: Experts Say the Trump Administration's Coronavirus Response Was Never Going to Work." *Time*, March 5, 2020. https://www.msn.com/en-au/news/world /doomed-from-the-start-experts-say-the-trump-administrations-coronavirus -response-was-never-going-to-work/ar-BB10OmVE (accessed July 3, 2020).

12. Keith, T. (2020). "Timeline: What Trump Has Said and Done about the Coronavirus." NPR, April 21, 2020. https://www.npr.org/2020/04/21/837348551 /timeline-what-trump-has-said-and-done-about-the-coronavirus (accessed July 4, 2020).

13. Bolton, *The Room Where It Happened.*

14. Bergengruen and Hennigan, "Doomed from the Start."

15. Ibid.

16. Ibid.

17. Ibid.

18. Villarreal, A. (2020). "Four Months and 100,000 Deaths" The Defining COVID-19 Moments in the U.S. Timeline." *The Guardian*, May 28, 2020. https://

www.theguardian.com/us-news/2020/apr/25/us-coronavirus-timeline-trump
-cases-deaths (accessed July 7, 2020).

19. Zamarripa, R. (2020). "5 Ways the Trump Administration's Policy Failures Compounded the Coronavirus-Induced Economic Crisis." Center for American Progress, June 3, 2020. https://www.americanprogress.org/issues/economy/news/2020/06/03/485806/5-ways-trump-administrations-policy-failures-compounded-coronavirus-induced-economic-crisis/ (accessed July 7, 2020).

20. Ibid.

21. Bendix, A. (2020). "The US's Failed Coronavirus Response Continues to Snowball—Even as Federal Officials Insist They're 'Winning the Fight.'" Business Insider, June 23, 2020. https://www.businessinsider.com/us-failed-coronavirus-response-reopening-exacerbated-first-wave-2020-6 (accessed July 7, 2020).

22. Levensen, E. (2020). "Why New York Is the Epicenter of the American Coronavirus Outbreak." CNN, March 26, 2020. https://www.cnn.com/2020/03/26/us/new-york-coronavirus-explainer/index.html (accessed July 9, 2020).

23. Ibid.

24. Scher, B. (2020). "Coronavirus vs. Governors: Ranking the Best and Worst State Leaders." Politico, April 1, 2020. https://www.politico.com/news/magazine/2020/04/01/coronavirus-state-governors-best-worst-covid-19-159945 (accessed July 9, 2020).

25. Ibid.

26. Ibid.

27. Ibid.

28. Ibid.

29. Ibid.

30. Ibid.

31. Pew Research Center. (2020). "Republicans, Democrats Move Even Further Apart in Coronavirus Concerns." June 25, 2020. https://www.pewresearch.org/politics/2020/06/25/republicans-democrats-move-even-further-apart-in-coronavirus-concerns/ (accessed July 12, 2020).

32. Kluch, S. (2020). "The Compliance Curve: Will People Stay Home Much Longer?" Gallup, April 29, 2020. https://news.gallup.com/opinion/gallup/309491/compliance-curve-americans-stay-home-covid.aspx (accessed July 12, 2020).

33. Jacobson, L., and McCarthy, B. (2020). "Large Majorities of Americans Support Keeping Stay-at-Home Policies for Now." Politico, April 22, 2020. https://www.politifact.com/article/2020/apr/22/large-majorities-americans-support-keeping-stay-ho/ (accessed July 13, 2020).

34. Ibid.

35. Ibid.

36. World Health Organization. (2020). "Coronavirus Disease (COVID-19) Pandemic." July 12, 2020. https://www.who.int/emergencies/diseases/novel-coronavirus-2019 (accessed July 13, 2020).

37. Smith, D. (2020). "Trump Calls Protesters against Stay-at-Home Orders 'Very Responsible.'" *The Guardian*, April 17, 2020. https://www.theguardian

.com/us-news/2020/apr/17/trump-liberate-tweets-coronavirus-stay-at-home
-orders (accessed July 13, 2020).

38. Ibid.

39. Aratani, L. (2020). "Jobless America: The Coronavirus Unemployment Crisis in Figures." *The Guardian*, May 28, 2020. https://www.theguardian.com /business/2020/may/28/jobless-america-unemployment-coronavirus-in-figures (accessed July 13, 2020).

40. H.R.6201. Families First Coronavirus Response Act. https://www.congress .gov/bill/116th-congress/house-bill/6201/text (accessed July 13, 2020).

41. S.3548. CARES Act. https://www.congress.gov/bill/116th-congress/senate -bill/3548 (accessed July 13, 2020).

42. Stewart, M. (2020). "The PPP Worked How It Was Supposed To. That's the Problem." Vox, July 13, 2020. https://www.vox.com/recode/2020/7/13/21320179 /ppp-loans-sba-paycheck-protection-program-polling-kanye-west (accessed July 14, 2020).

43. Ibid.

44. Romano, A. (2020). "A New Investigation Reveals Trump Ignored Experts on COVID-19 for Months." Vox, April 12, 2020. https://www.vox .com/2020/4/12/21218305/trump-ignored-coronavirus-warnings (accessed July 14, 2020).

45. Ibid.

46. Ibid.

47. Schneider, R.O. (2018). *When Science and Politics Collide: The Public Interest at Risk*. Santa Barbara, CA: Praeger.

48. Gordon, R. (2020). "Why Can't I Stop Watching Trump's Chaotic Briefings?" *The Nation*, April 21, 2020. www.thenation.com/article/politics/trump -press-briefings/ (accessed July 15, 2020).

49. Cathey, L. (2020). "Trump versus the Doctors: When the President and His Experts Contradict Each Other." ABC News, April 24, 2020. https://abcnews .go.com/Politics/trump-versus-doctors-president-experts-contradict/story? id=70330642 (accessed July 16, 2020).

50. Lysol. (2020). "Coronavirus." https://www.lysol.com/en/healthy-home /understanding-coronavirus/ (accessed July 16, 2020).

51. Peters, J.W., Plott, E., and Haberman, M. (2020). "260,000 Words, Full of Self-Praise, from Trump on the Virus. *New York Times*, April 27, 2020. https:// www.nytimes.com/interactive/2020/04/26/us/politics/trump-coronavirus -briefings-analyzed.html (accessed July 16, 2020).

52. Berlinger, J., Renton, A., and Reynolds, E. (2020). "June 1 Coronavirus News." CNN, June 1, 2020. https://www.cnn.com/world/live-news/coronavirus -pandemic-06-01-20-intl/index.html (accessed July 16, 2020).

53. Pei, S., Sasikiran, K., and Shaman, J. (2020). "Differential Effects of Intervention Timing on COVID-19 Spread in the United States." MedRxiv. https:// www.medrxiv.org/content/10.1101/2020.05.15.20103655v2 (accessed July 17, 2020).

Chapter Five

1. Bahar, D. (2020). "Reopening America: A Review of Metrics to Help Decision-Makers Determine the Proper Pace of Reopening." Brookings Institute, June 24, 2020. https://www.brookings.edu/blog/up-front/2020/06/24/reopening-america-a-review-of-metrics-to-help-decision-makers-determine-the-proper-pace-of-reopening/(accessed July 21, 2020).

2. Romer, P. (2020). "Roadmap to Responsibly Reopen America." Paulromer.net. https://paulromer.net/roadmap-to-reopen-america/ (accessed July 21, 2020).

3. Hausman, R. (2020). "Target R and Wait for the Vaccine." Project Syndicate, April 23, 2020. https://www.project-syndicate.org/commentary/target-covid19-infection-rate-for-restarting-economies-by-ricardo-hausmann-2020-04 (accessed July 21, 2020).

4. NPR. (2020). "President Trump Wants to Reopen Economy despite CDC Warnings." May 6, 2020. https://www.npr.org/2020/05/06/851631806/president-trump-wants-to-reopen-economy-despite-cdc-warnings (accessed July 22, 2020).

5. Cassidy, J. (2020). "The White House's Push to Reopen the Economy This Early Is a Dangerous Gamble." *New Yorker*, May 5, 2020. https://www.newyorker.com/news/our-columnists/the-white-houses-push-to-reopen-the-economy-this-early-is-a-dangerous-gamble (accessed July 22, 2020).

6. Gstalter, M. (2020). "White House Shelved CDC Reopening Guidance: Report." The Hill, May 7, 2020. https://thehill.com/homenews/administration/496528-white-house-shelved-cdc-reopening-guidance-report (accessed July 23, 2020).

7. Dearen, J. (2020). "Trump Administration Shelves CDC Guidance on How to Reopen Country." KSL.com, May 7, 2020. https://www.ksl.com/article/46750402/trump-administration-buries-detailed-cdc-advice-on-reopening (accessed July 19, 2021).

8. CDC. (2020). "Opening Up America Again." https://trumpwhitehouse.archives.gov/wp-content/uploads/2020/04/Guidelines-for-Opening-Up-America-Again.pdf (accessed July 23, 2020).

9. Ibid.

10. Lopez, G. (2020). "Just 3 States Meet These Basic Criteria to Reopen and Stay Safe." Vox, May 28, 2020. https://www.vox.com/2020/5/28/21270515/coronavirus-covid-reopen-economy-social-distancing-states-map-data (accessed July 23, 2020).

11. Samuels, A. (2020). "Dan Patrick Says 'There Are More Important Things Than Living and That's Saving This Country.'" *Texas Tribune*, April 21, 2020. https://www.texastribune.org/2020/04/21/texas-dan-patrick-economy-coronavirus/ (accessed July 24, 2020).

12. Edwards, H.S. (2020). "There Are Sensible Ways to Reopen a Country. Then There's America's Approach." *Time*, May 14, 2020. https://time.com/5836607/reopening-risks-coronavirus/ (accessed July 24, 2020).

13. Ibid.

14. Ibid.

15. Ibid.

16. Ibid.

17. Newkirk, M. (2020). "Georgia Massaged Virus Data to Reopen, Then Voided Mask Orders." Bloomberg, July 17, 2020. https://www.bloomberg.com /news/articles/2020-07-17/georgia-massaged-virus-data-to-reopen-then-voided -mask-orders (accessed July 28, 2020).

18. Ibid.

19. Benen, S. (2020). "DeSantis' Response Panned as 'Divorced from Scientific Evidence.'" MSNBC, July 27, 2020. https://www.msnbc.com/rachel-maddow -show/desantis-response-panned-divorced-scientific-evidence-n1234959 (accessed July 28, 2020).

20. Wootson, C.R., Stanley-Becker, I., Rozsa, L., and Dawsey, J. (2020). "Coronavirus Ravaged Florida, as Ron DeSantis Sidelined Scientists and Followed Trump." *Washington Post*, July 25, 2020. https://www.washingtonpost.com /national/coronavirus-ravaged-florida-as-ron-desantis-sidelined-scientists-and -followed-trump/2020/07/25/0b8008da-c648-11ea-b037-f9711f89ee46_story .html (accessed July 28, 2020).

21. Platoff, E. (2020). "A Singular Figure in Texas' Coronavirus Response, Gov. Greg Abbott Leads a State Headed in an Alarming Direction." *Texas Tribune*, July 11, 2020. https://www.texastribune.org/2020/07/11/texas-greg-abbott-coronavirus -response/ (accessed July 30, 2020).

22. Ibid.

23. Sainato, M. (2020). "Texas Hospital Forced to Set Up 'Death Panel' as COVID-19 Cases Surge." *The Guardian*, July 26, 2020. https://www.theguardian .com/world/2020/jul/26/covid-19-death-panels-starr-county-hospital-texas (accessed July 30, 2020).

24. Roberts, L. (2020). "Gov. Doug Ducey Fires the Scientists Who Warn He's Making a Mistake by Reopening Arizona." *Arizona Republic*, May 6, 2020. https:// www.azcentral.com/story/opinion/op-ed/laurieroberts/2020/05/06/arizona-not -ready-reopen-asu-ua-coronavirus-models-say-fired/5175510002/ (accessed July 30, 2020).

25. Berryman, K., and Waldrop, T. (2020). "Arizona Closes Bars, Gyms and Other Businesses after 'Brutal' Increase in COVID-19 Cases." CNN, June 30, 2020. https://edition.cnn.com/2020/06/29/us/arizona-covid-19-closures/index .html (accessed July 30, 2020).

26. Rong-Gong, L., Blume, H., Gutierrez, M. Fry, H., and Dolan, M. (2020). "How California Went from a Rapid Reopening to a Second Closing in One Month." *Los Angeles Times*, July 14, 2020. https://www.latimes.com/california /story/2020-07-14/california-reopening-shutdown-coronavirus-spike (accessed July 30, 2020).

27. Budryk, Z. (2020). "21 States Now in Federal 'Red Zone' for Serious Coronavirus Outbreaks: Study." The Hill, July 28, 2020. https://thehill.com/policy /healthcare/509418-21-states-now-in-federal-red-zone-for-serious-coronavirus -outbreaks-report (accessed July 30, 2020).

28. Igielink, R. (2020). "Most Americans Say They Regularly Wore a Mask in Stores in the Past Month; Fewer See Others Doing It." Pew Research Center, June 23, 2020. https://www.pewresearch.org/fact-tank/2020/06/23/most-americans-say-they-regularly-wore-a-mask-in-stores-in-the-past-month-fewer-see-others-doing-it/ (accessed August 6, 2020).

29. Ibid.

30. Jackson, C., and Newall, M. (2020). "Social Distancing Diminishes as Americans Increasingly Rely on Masks." Ipsos, August 4, 2020. https://www.ipsos.com/en-us/news-polls/axios-ipsos-coronavirus-index (accessed August 6, 2020).

31. Ibid.

32. Rubin, T. (2020). "President Trump's Promotion of 'Demon Sperm' Dr. Stella Immanuel Bodes Ill for Second Term." *Philadelphia Inquirer*, August 1, 2020.

33. Forgey, Q., and Oprysko, C. (2020). "I Happen to Think It Works: Trump Doubles Down on Hydroxychloroquine." Politico, July 28, 2020. https://www.msn.com/en-us/news/politics/fauci-rebukes-trump-s-renewed-push-for-ineffective-covid-19-treatment/ar-BB17hqQZ (accessed July 19, 2021).

34. Farzan, A.N., Noack, R., O'Grady, S., Shammas, B., Knowles, H., Bellwatre, K., and Shaban, H. (2020). "Live Updates: Nearly 100,000 U.S. Children Test Positive for Coronavirus in Two-Week Span." *Washington Post*, August 10, 2020. https://www.washingtonpost.com/nation/2020/08/10/coronavirus-covid-live-updates-us/ (accessed August 10, 2020).

35. Ibid.

36. Global Health Security Index. (2019). "2019 Global Health Security Index." www.ghsindex.org (accessed August 10, 2020).

37. Ibid.

Chapter Six

1. Arnold, C. (2020). "Why the U.S. Coronavirus Testing Failures Were Inevitable." *National Geographic*, March 30, 2020.

2. Schneider, E.C. (2020). "Failing the Test: The Tragic Data Gap Undermining the U.S. Pandemic Response." *New England Journal of Medicine* 383: 299–302.

3. Rosenthal, E. (2020). "Analysis: We Knew the Coronavirus Was Coming, Yet We Failed 5 Critical Tests." *New York Times*, May 11, 2020.

4. Yglesias, M. (2020). "Trump's Catastrophic Failure on Testing Is No Joke." Vox, June 23, 2020 (accessed September 8, 2020).

5. Todd, C., Murray, M., Dann, C., and Holzberg, M. (2020). "Trump again Downplays Coronavirus with Indoor Campaign Rally." *Meet the Press*, September 14, 2020. https://www.nbcnews.com/politics/meet-the-press/trump-again-downplays-coronavirus-indoor-campaign-rally-n1240008 (accessed September 17, 2020).

6. Woodward, B. (2020). *Rage*. New York: Simon and Schuster.

7. Ibid.

8. Ibid.

9. Ibid.

10. Armed Conflict Location and Event Data Project. (2020). "Demonstrations and Political Violence in America: New Data for Summer 2020." https://acleddata.com/2020/09/03/demonstrations-political-violence-in-america-new-data-for-summer-2020/ (accessed September 21, 2020).

11. Ibid.

12. Ibid.

13. Woodward, *Rage*.

14. Wilson, R. (2020). "Despair at CDC after Trump Influence: 'I Have Never Seen Morale This Low.'" The Hill, September 23, 2020. https://thehill.com/policy/healthcare/517708-despair-at-cdc-after-trump-influence-i-have-never-seen-morale-this-low (accessed September 24, 2020).

15. Ibid.

16. Heavy.com. (2020). "Dr. Scott Atlas: Trump's New Coronavirus Adviser Backs Him on Schools & Sport." https://heavy.com/news/2020/08/scott-atlas/ (accessed September 30, 2020).

17. NBCU. (2020). "CDC Director on Dr. Scott Atlas: 'Everything He Says Is False.'" https://news.yahoo.com/cdc-director-dr-scott-atlas-213555944.html (accessed October 1, 2020).

18. Nierenberg, A., and Pasick, A. (2020). "Schools Briefing: The Outlook for In-Person Classes." *New York Times*, August 24, 2020. https://www.nytimes.com/2020/08/24/us/college-university-reopening-coronavirus.html (accessed October 7, 2020).

19. Ibid.

20. Ibid.

21. Courage, K.A. (2020). "Why Some Colleges Are Winning against COVID-19 and Others Are Losing." Vox, October 10, 2020. https://www.vox.com/21445908/covid-19-prevention-university-campus-dorms-testing (accessed October 13, 2020).

22. Ibid.

23. North, A. (2020). "10 Facts about Reopening in the COVID-19 Pandemic." Vox, October 1, 2020. https://www.vox.com/2020/10/1/21493602/covid-19-schools-reopening-nyc-florida-hybrid (accessed October 15, 2020).

24. Education Week. (2020). "Map: Where Are Schools Closed?" October 16, 2020. https://www.edweek.org/ew/section/multimedia/map-covid-19-schools-open-closed.html (accessed October 20, 2020).

25. Lopez, G. (2020). "What We've Learned So Far from School Reopenings in the U.S." Vox, October 16, 2020. https://www.vox.com/future-perfect/21494352/school-reopenings-covid-coronavirus-pandemic-in-person-teaching (accessed October 20, 2020).

26. Ibid.

27. Associated Press. (2020). "School Reopenings Linked to Coronavirus Cases among U.S. Children." *Oregonian*, September 29, 2020. https://www

.oregonlive.com/coronavirus/2020/09/school-reopenings-linked-to-increase-in
-coronavirus-cases-among-us-children.html) (accessed October 20, 2020).

28. Housman, D. (2020). "School Reopenings Haven't Led to COVID-19 Outbreaks Yet, According to Early Evidence." Daily Caller, September 23, 2020.
https://dailycaller.com/2020/09/23/brown-university-reopening-schools-covid
-outbreaks/ (accessed October 20, 2020).

29. Maxouris, C., and Yan, H. (2020). "Hunker Down: The Fall COVID-19
Surge Is Here." CNN, October 13, 2020. https://www.cnn.com/2020/10/13
/health/us-coronavirus-tuesday/index.html (accessed October 27, 2020).

30. Ibid.

31. Sheinin, A.G. (2020). "Trump Leaves Hospital after COVID Treatment."
WebMD, October 5, 2020. https://www.webmd.com/lung/news/20201004
/trump-could-be-released-from-hospital-monday (accessed October 28, 2020).

32. Ibid.

33. Lyons, G. (2020). "Trump Super-Spreader Events Are Immoral and Criminal." *Chicago Sun-Times*, October 28, 2020. https://chicago.suntimes.com
/columnists/2020/10/28/21539209/trump-maga-rally-super-spreaders-typhoid
-mary-gene-lyons (accessed November 2, 2020).

34. Wong, W., Sheeley, C., and Siemaszko, C. (2020). "Once again, U.S.
Records New Daily High, Nearly 100,000, for COVID-19 Cases." NBC News,
October 30, 2020. https://www.nbcnews.com/news/us-news/u-s-records-more
-90-000-covid-19-cases-one-n1245450 (accessed November 2, 2020).

35. CDC COVID Data Tracker. (2020). https://covid.cdc.gov/covid-data
-tracker/#cases_casesinlast7days (accessed November 2, 2020).

36. The Harris Poll COVID-19 Portal. (2020). https://mailchi.mp/58a325d432f5
/the-insight-latest-trends-from-the-harris-poll-304670 (accessed November 3, 2020).

37. Rosen, D. (2020). "After COVID: Will Recession Become a Depression."
Counterpunch, October 28, 2020. https://www.counterpunch.org/2020/10/28
/after-covid-will-the-recession-become-a-depression/ (accessed November 9, 2020).

38. U.S. Department of Labor. (2020). "News Release." November 5, 2020.
https://www.dol.gov/ui/data.pdf (accessed November 9, 2020).

39. Congressional Research Service. (2020). "Unemployment Rates during
the COVID-19 Pandemic." November 6, 2020. https://crsreports.congress.gov
/product/pdf/R/R46554 (accessed November 9, 2020).

40. Bredemeir, K. (2020). "Fauci: US Economy Won't Recover until Coronavirus Controlled." VOA News, April 20, 2020. https://www.voanews.com/covid
-19-pandemic/fauci-us-economy-wont-recover-until-coronavirus-controlled
(accessed November 9, 2020).

41. H.R.6800. The Heroes Act. https://www.congress.gov/bill/116th-congress
/house-bill/6800 (accessed November 17, 2020).

42. Klebnikov, S. (2020). "Republicans Appalled by $3 Trillion Heroes Acts as
Democrats Urge Its Passing." *Forbes*, May 16, 2020. https://www.forbes.com
/sites/sergeiklebnikov/2020/05/16/republicans-appalled-by-3-trillion-heroes-act
-as-democrats-urge-its-passing/ (accessed November 17, 2020).

43. NPR Staff. (2020). "Understanding the 2020 Electorate: AP VoteCast Survey." NPR.org, November 3, 2020. https://www.npr.org/2020/11/03/929478378 /understanding-the-2020-electorate-ap-votecast-survey (accessed November 24, 2020).

44. Fung, M. (2020). "COVID-19 Cases Surge around the World amid Fears the Worst Is Yet to Come." *Straits Times*, November 13, 2020. https://www.straitstimes .com/world/covid-19-cases-surge-around-the-world-amid-fears-the-worst-is-yet -to-come (accessed November 30, 2020).

45. Schwartz, M.S. (2020). "Fauci Warns of Surge upon Surge as COVID-19 Hospitalizations Hit Yet Another High." NPR, November 30, 2020. https://www.wbez .org/stories/fauci-warns-of-surge-upon-a-surge-as-covid-19-hospitalizations-hit-yet -another-high/ab641285-0399-4dd6-aa90-9ceed844e457 (accessed November 30, November 30, 2020).

Chapter Seven

1. Harris Poll. (2020). "Yahoo Finance/The Harris Poll: Americans Divided on COVID-19 Vaccine." https://theharrispoll.com/americans-divided-covid-vaccine -fda/ (accessed December 22, 2020).

2. Goldstein, A. (2020). "Biden Lays Out Plan to Combat COVID in First 100 Days, Including Requiring Masks on Interstate Buses, Trains." *Washington Post*, December 8, 2020. https://www.washingtonpost.com/health/biden-covid-100 -days-plan/2020/12/08/16e0a47e-3965-11eb-98c4-25dc9f4987e8_story.html (accessed December 28, 2020).

3. Halper, E., and Levey, N. (2020). "'Wear a Mask': Biden Urges Coronavirus Caution as He Praises Vaccine Progress." *Los Angeles Times*, November 9, 2020.

4. Ibid.

5. Evelyn, K. (2020). "Fauci Accepts Offer of Chief Medical Adviser Role in Biden Administration." *The Guardian*, December 4, 2020. https://www.theguardian.com /us-news/2020/dec/04/fauci-accepts-biden-offer-chief-medical-adviser (accessed December 28, 2020).

6. Collinson, S. (2020). "Trump's Transition Sabotage Threatens COVID-19 Vaccine Rollout." CNN, November 17, 2020. https://www.msn.com/en-us/news /politics/trump-s-transition-sabotage-threatens-vaccine-rollout/ar-BB1b4EXy (accessed December 30, 2020).

7. Heer, J. (2020). "Trump's Team Is Sabotaging the Transition." *The Nation*, November 25, 2020. https://www.thenation.com/article/politics/trump-sabotage -transition-biden (accessed December 30, 2020).

8. Ibid.

9. Wingrove, J. (2020). "Trump Is Silent on Record Virus Deaths as He Fumes over Loss." Bloomberg, December 3, 2020. https://www.bloomberg.com/news /articles/2020-12-03/trump-silent-on-virus-despite-record-hospitalizations -deaths (accessed January 4, 2021).

10. Healthline. (2020). "Here Are the States Where COVID-19 Is Increasing." https://www.healthline.com/health-news/here-are-the-states-where-covid-19-is-increasing (accessed January 6, 2021).

11. Institute for Health Metrics and Evaluation (IHME). (2021). "COVID-10 Projections." https://covid19.healthdata.org/united-states-of-america?view=total-deaths&tab=trend (accessed January 6, 2021).

12. Colliver, V.I. (2020). "Locked-Down California Runs Out of Reasons for Surprising Surge." *Los Angeles Times*, December 23, 2020. https://www.politico.com/news/2020/12/23/california-covid-surge-450315 (accessed January 6, 2021).

13. Associated Press. (2021). "Nearly a Third of Alabama's COVID Cases Came in December: 'We Are Going to See Even Worse Numbers'" AL.com, January 1, 2021. https://www.al.com/news/2021/01/nearly-a-third-of-alabamas-covid-cases-came-in-december-we-are-going-to-see-even-worse-numbers.html (accessed January 6, 2021).

14. Mack, Z. (2020). "This State Now Has the Worst COVID Outbreak in the U.S." Bestlifeonline. https://bestlifeonline.com/tennessee-covid-2/ (accessed January 6, 2021).

15. Evans, M. (2021) "'It's a Desperate Time': Crush of COVID-19 Patients Strains U.S. Hospitals." *Wall Street Journal*, January 4, 2021. https://www.msn.com/en-us/health/medical/its-a-desperate-time-crush-of-covid-19-patients-strains-us-hospitals/ar-BB1cre0E (accessed January 6, 2021).

16. Coleman, K. (2020). "Dr. Fauci Just Made a Scary Admission about the COVID Surge." Bestlifeonline, December 29, 2020. https://bestlifeonline.com/fauci-scary-covid-surge/ (accessed January 8, 2021).

17. Quinn, J. (2020). "Dr. Fauci Just Said These 3 Things Are about to Make COVID Worse." Bestlifeonline, December 27, 2020. https://bestlifeonline.com/fauci-covid-worse/ (accessed January 8, 2021).

18. Palus, S. (2021). "America Is Failing at the Boring Part." Slate, January 5, 2021. https://slate.com/technology/2021/01/vaccine-failing-at-the-boring-part.html (accessed January 12, 2021).

19. Ibid.

20. Murphy, J., and Siemaszko, C. (2020). "Operation Warp Speed at a Crawl: Adequately Vaccinating Americans Will Take 10 Years at Current Pace." NBC News, December 30, 2020. https://www.cnbc.com/2020/12/30/operation-warp-speed-at-a-crawl-adequately-vaccinating-americans-will-take-10-years-at-current-pace.html (accessed January 12, 2021).

21. Bollinger, R. (2021). "A New Strain of Coronavirus: What You Should Know." Johns Hopkins Medicine. https://www.hopkinsmedicine.org/health/conditions-and-diseases/coronavirus/a-new-strain-of-coronavirus-what-you-should-know (accessed January 12, 2021).

22. Ibid.

23. Henley, J. (2021). "Europe at Tipping Point with COVID Running Rampant, Says WHO." *The Guardian*, January 7, 2021. https://www.theguardian.com/world/2021/jan/07/europe-tipping-point-covid-running-rampant-who-new-variant (accessed January 12, 2021).

24. Garrett, A. (2021). "New, More Transmissible COVID Strain Found in These States." *Newsweek*, January 4, 2021. https://www.newsweek.com/new-more-transmissible-covid-strain-found-these-states-1558851 (accessed January 12, 2021).

25. Steib, M. (2021). "New COVID Strain Spreading across U.S.: What We Know." *New York*, February 7, 2021. https://nymag.com/intelligencer/article/what-is-the-new-covid-19-strain-that-shut-down-england-u-k.html (accessed January 12, 2021).

26. Gander, K. (2021). "U.S COVID Death Toll Could Hit 477,000 by Early February, CDC Says." *Newsweek*, January 14, 2021. https://www.msn.com/en-us/news/us/us-covid-death-toll-could-hit-477000-by-early-february-cdc-says/ar-BB1cL0iO (accessed January 14, 2021).

27. Dale, D. (2020). "Fact Checking Trump's Barrage of Lies over the Weekend." CNN, November 16, 2020. https://www.cnn.com/2020/11/16/politics/fact-check-trump-rigged-election-dominion-georgia-pennsylvania/index.html (accessed January 18, 2021).

28. Ibid.

29. Cummings, W., Garrison, J., and Sergent, J. (2021). "Trump and Allies Filed Scores of Lawsuits, Tried to Convince State Legislatures to Take Action, Organized Protests and Held Hearings. . . . None of It Worked." *USA Today*, January 6, 2021. https://www.usatoday.com/in-depth/news/politics/elections/2021/01/06/trumps-failed-efforts-overturn-election-numbers/4130307001/ (accessed January 18, 2021).

30. Pew Research Center. (2021). "Voters' Reflections on the 2020 Election." Survey, January 15, 2021. https://www.pewresearch.org/politics/2021/01/15/voters-reflections-on-the-2020-election/ (accessed January 19, 2021).

31. Sher, M.D., and Kanno-Youngs, Z. (2020). "In Arizona, Trump Boasts about His Wall and Repeats Unfounded Predictions of Voter Fraud." *New York Times*, June 23, 2020. https://www.nytimes.com/2020/06/23/us/politics/trump-arizona.html (accessed January 19, 2021).

32. Fearnow, B. (2020). "Trump Encourages 'Wild' Protests in D.C. on Date of Electoral College Vote Count." *Newsweek*, December 19, 2020. https://www.msn.com/en-us/news/politics/trump-encourages-wild-protests-in-d-c-on-date-of-electoral-college-vote-count/ar-BB1c4nn9 (accessed January 21, 2021).

33. Trump, D. (2021). "Donald Trump Speech 'Save America' Rally Transcript January 6." Rev, January 6, 2021. https://www.rev.com/blog/transcripts/donald-trump-speech-save-america-rally-transcript-january-6 (accessed January 21, 2021).

34. Petras, G., Loehrke, J., Padilla, R., Zarracina, J. and Borresen, J. (2021). "Timeline: How a Trump Mob Stormed the US Capitol, Forcing Washington into Lockdown." *USA Today*, January 15, 2021. https://www.usatoday.com/in-depth /news/2021/01/06/dc-protests-capitol-riot-trump-supporters-electoral-college -stolen-election/6568305002/ (accessed January dep21, 2021).

35. Ibid.

36. Ibid.

Index

Page numbers followed by a "t" represent tables in the book.

Centers for Disease Control and
Prevention (CDC), vii, 2, 24, 26,
45, 67, 74, 108, 138, 173; and
COVID guidelines, 26–27, 30–31,
108; "reopening" guidelines, 109;
and White House interference with,
109–110
Challenges to the 2020 election
results, 167–169, 176–179,
185–197
Conspiracy theories, 54, 66, 120–123,
166, 177–178
Containment strategy, 77–78, 102
Cooper, Roy, 115
Coronavirus, 5–8; types, 4, 72; and
voters in the 2020 election,
166–167
COVID-19 mutations, 172–173
COVID-19 symptoms and stages,
5–6
COVID treatments, vii, 7, 10, 31, 67,
77, 80, 99, 107, 120, 128–129,
139, 147, 156, 182
Cuomo, Andrew, 81–82, 98–99; daily
press briefings, 82
Cybersecurity and Infrastructure
Security Agency, 186

de Blasio, Bill, 81–82
Department of Health and Human
Services, 8, 35, 45, 67, 80, 138
Department of Homeland Security
(DHS), 28, 39
DeSantis, Ron, 84, 117
DeWine, Mike, 83
Diaz, George, vii
Dominion Voting Systems, 185
Ducey, Doug, 118, 119
Dzau, Victor, 40

Ebola epidemic, 37–38, 40
Economic impacts of COVID-19,
92–95
Eisenhower, Dwight, 43, 46

Election Day 2020, 108, 158,
164–166, 168
Electoral College, 167, 186–187, 189
Electoral College certification in
Congress, 187, 189
Epidemics, 4, 8, 29, 31, 33, 37
Ethical dimension of a pandemic
threat, 34

Families First Coronavirus Act, 93
Failures, 10, 34, 38, 40, 72, 99, 138,
141, 174, 183, 194–195, 197
Fauci, Anthony, 64, 97, 113, 146,
162, 168–169, 180, 183; and
Congressional testimony, 113,
122–123; and the experts *versus*
Trump, 146–148; and Joe Biden,
175; and public trust in experts,
55–56
Federal Drug Administration (FDA),
148, 172
Financial crisis of 2008, 20
First American COVID-19 death, 16
First wave: the global timeline, 12–18
Floyd, George, 143–144

Galileo, 50
General Services Administration
(GSA), 176
Giuliani, Rudy, 188
Global Health (GHS) Security Index,
131, 192
Governors respond, 79–86

Herd immunity, 172, 197
HEROES Act, 162–163, 184
H5N1 pandemic threat, 27–28; H5N1
planning process, 33–37; H5N1
and the Bush administration, 23–24
Hicks, Hope, 155
H1N1 pandemic, 34–37, 46, 174
H1N1 vaccine development, 36
Hofstadter, Richard, 53
Hogan, Larry, 84

About the Author

Robert O. Schneider, PhD, is a political scientist with expertise in the field of emergency management. Much of his research focuses on disaster mitigation and sustainability. He has also researched and written on leading policy issues where science and politics intersect. He is the author of Praeger's *When Science and Politics Collide: The Public Interest at Risk* (2018) and *Managing the Climate Crisis: Assessing Our Risks, Options, and Prospects* (2015).